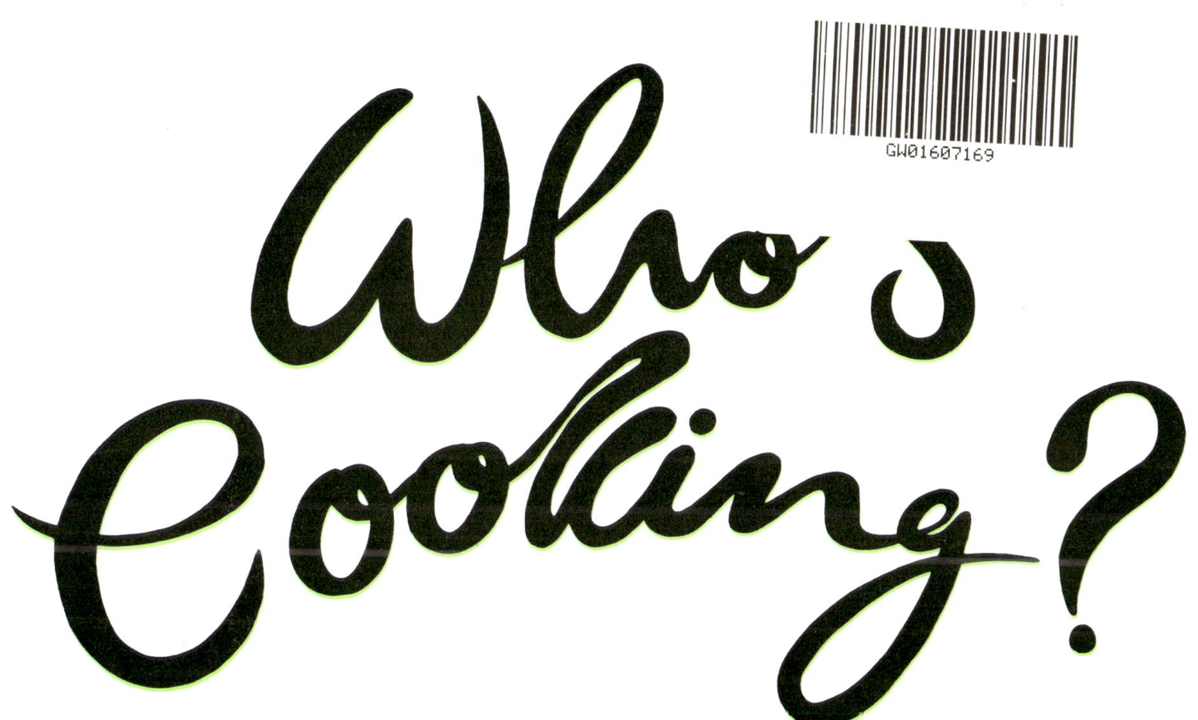
Who's
Cooking?
GW01607169

Alzheimer's Disease Society
158-160 Balham High Road
London SW12 9BN
Tel: 081-675 6557

Charity no. 296645
Limited by Guarantee
Registered no. 2115499

Published: October 1991
ISBN 1 872874 08 8

Contents

Introduction

The original idea for this cookery book was to produce a collection of recipes for carers who need meals which are either quick or easy to prepare, whether for every day or for special occasions.

We then thought of including recipes from celebrities to add an extra sparkle to the pages. The response from the celebrities we approached was overwhelming, and we thank every one of them. We must also thank everybody else – particularly our hard-pressed carers – who contributed to the book. We are only sorry that we were unable to include every recipe – we simply didn't have room. Each chapter has a 'Quick or Easy' section to tie in with the original purpose of helping carers with their 24 hour-a-day task.

Our final "thank-you's" must be to Ann Blofield, a volunteer who spent many hours helping me to compile the book, and to Tracy Deekes, the talented artist who illustrated it. Alas, we could not cook every recipe, so cannot absolutely attest to each one!

Thank you for buying this book and contributing to the Society's much needed funds. May you enjoy many happy and tasty meals as a result of your generosity.

PAULA DAWE
Appeals Officer

Metric Measures

Mass

1 ounce	=	30 grams	1 pound	=	500 grams
4 ounces	=	125 grams	2 pounds	=	1kg
8 ounces	=	250 grams	5 pounds	=	2.5 kg

Liquids

¼ teaspoon	=	1 ml.	¼ cup	=	60 mls.
½ teaspoon	=	2 mls.	⅓ cup	=	80 mls.
1 teaspoon	=	5 mls.	½ cup	=	125 mls.
1 tablespoon	=	12.5 mls.	1 cup	=	250 mls.

Other Volumes

1 pint	=	600 mls	3 pints	=	1.90 litres
2 pints	=	1.25 litres	4 pints	=	2.50 litres

Oven Temperatures (approx.)

		175°F	=	80°C
		200°F	=	90°C
¼-½ (cool)	=	250°F	=	120°C
1	=	275°F	=	140°C
2	=	300°F	=	150°C
3	=	325°F	=	160°C
4 (mod.)	=	350°F	=	180°C
5	=	375°F	=	190°C
6	=	400°F	=	200°C
7 (hot)	=	425°F	=	220°C
8	=	450°F	=	230°C
9	=	475°F	=	250°C
		500°F	=	260°C

Measurements in this book are generally imperial. Please use conversion table for approximate metric equivalents.

Starters & Soups

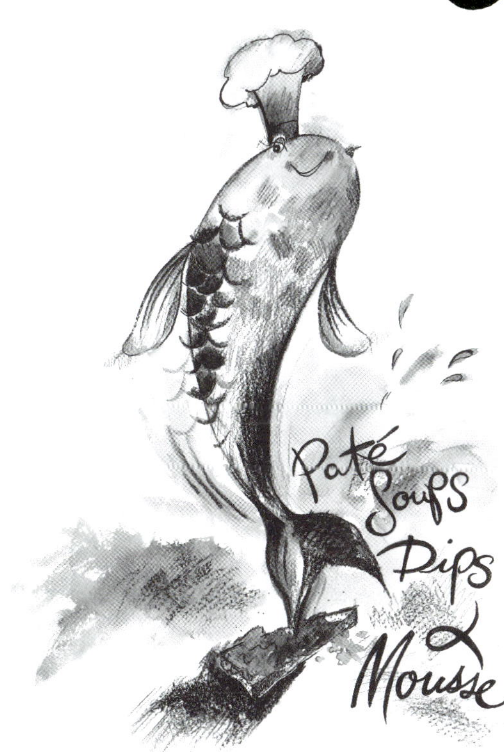

Kipper Paté

Ingredients

6oz kipper fillets
4oz cottage cheese
2oz melted butter

1 tablespoon lemon juice
1 tablespoon Worcester sauce
3 tablespoons melted butter
(for finish)

Method

Remove skin and any large bones from kippers.

Place kippers, cottage cheese, melted butter, lemon juice and Worcester sauce in blender. Liquidise.

Spoon into small dishes, seal with melted butter, chill and serve. Will freeze well.

Serves 6.

HER ROYAL HIGHNESS PRINCESS ALEXANDRA

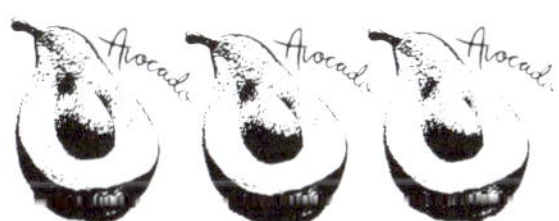

Avocado with Raspberry Vinaigrette

Ingredients

2 avocado pears, halved and stoned
1 tablespoon lemon juice
4oz raspberries
2 tablespoons olive oil
1 tablespoon wine vinegar
½ teaspoon clear honey
Salt and pepper
Fennel leaves to garnish (optional)

Method

Peel each avocado half and place cut side down on a serving plate. Slice through the avocados lengthways, then separate the slices slightly. Brush lightly with lemon juice.

Press the raspberries through a nylon sieve to remove the seeds, then mix with oil, vinegar, honey and salt and pepper to taste.

Spoon a little around each avocado pear and serve immediately, garnished with fennel.

Serves 4.

COLCHESTER STANWAY TOWNSWOMEN'S GUILD

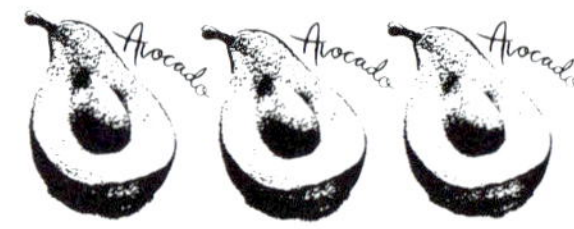

Lemon, Lime and Cottage Cheese Mould

Ingredients

1 packet of lime jelly
¾ pint hot water
1½ cups cottage cheese (8oz tub)
2 teaspoons lemon juice
¼ cup mayonnaise
1 small tin crushed pineapple (drained)
6 chopped glacé cherries

Method

Dissolve lime jelly in hot water. Leave until nearly set. Blend with cottage cheese, lemon juice and mayonnaise. Leave to set slightly. Add pineapple and cherries. Put into moulds and refrigerate.

Serve on lettuce leaves.

Comments

Many of the Nova Scotians are descendants of the original German settlers, who fought with the British in the American War of Independence and had to sail north when the British were defeated. There is therefore a German/American mixed origin to their food. This salad was given to me from an inhabitant of Lunenburg, a fishing town on the coast.

JOAN ALCOCK

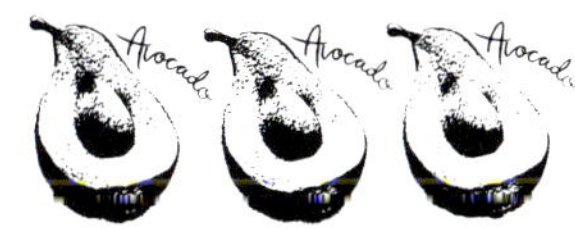

Mushrooms a la Greque

Ingredients

1 tablespoon oil
1 onion, diced
1 clove garlic, crushed
4 tablespoons tomato puree
¼ pint white wine or vermouth
1 teaspoon dried herbs
12oz button mushrooms
Salt and pepper to taste

Method

Cook the onion and oil in a large casserole dish in the microwave on high for 1 minute or until soft. Stir in other ingredients. Cover and cook on high for 5 more minutes or until the mushrooms are tender. Serve hot or chilled.

Serves 4.

VI WRIGHT
National Office, Alzheimer's Disease Society, Balham

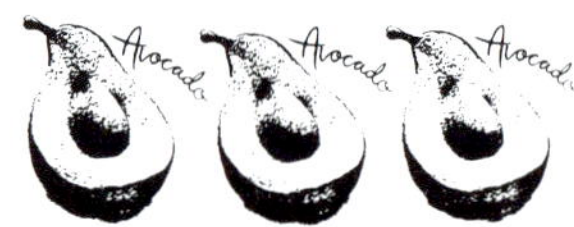

Sardine Mousse

Ingredients

1 tin sardines in oil, drained
1 small carton natural yoghurt
2 spring onions, chopped
3 inch chunk of cucumber, chopped
1 tablespoon lemon juice
Shake of pepper
¼oz (half a sachet) of gelatine dissolved in 2 tablespoons of boiling water

Method

Mix all the ingredients in a food processor until smooth (or mash them together if you do not have a processor for a 'rough' mixture). Pour into 2 or 4 appropriately-sized souffle dishes moistened with water. Chill until set. To remove, run a small palette knife around mousse, invert onto salad and gently shake and ease out.

Serve with a small salad and garnish with chives, olives, gherkins or capers.

Serves 2 if you are greedy and 4 if you are not!

MRS J. E. WILLIAMS
Mid-Sussex Branch

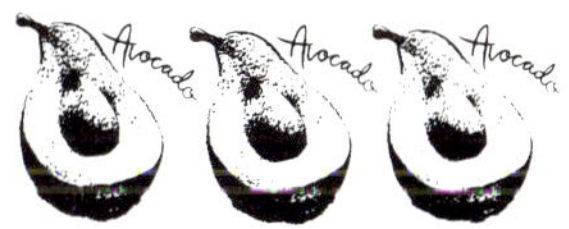

Little Ham Puffs

Ingredients

2oz flour
2 eggs
8oz finely chopped ham
Salt and pepper
Oil

Method

Separate the whites from the yolks and beat whites until stiff. Mix the flour with the egg yolks to a smooth paste. Fold in the whites, season and mix in the ham. Drop 1 teaspoon at a time into hot oil. Cook until light brown.

Drain well and serve either hot or cold.

COLCHESTER STANWAY TOWNSWOMEN'S GUILD

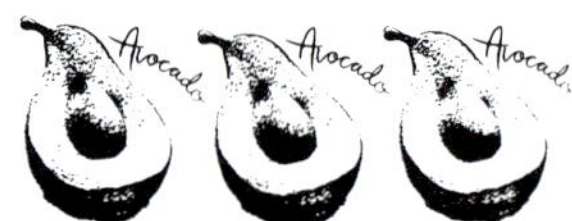

Borsch

Ingredients

½ cup carrots
1 cup onions
1 cup raw beetroot
1 tablespoon butter/margarine
2 cups beef stock
1 cup tomato pulp or puree
1 cup finely shredded cabbage

Method

Peel carrots, onions and beetroot and chop finely. Put them into a pan and barely cover with boiling water. Simmer covered for 20 minutes. Add butter/margarine, stock, tomato pulp or puree and cabbage. Boil for 15 minutes.

Serve hot or cold.

BILL BARTLETT
Buckinghamshire Branch

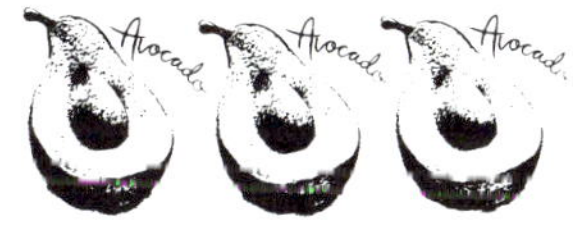

Leek and Potato Soup

Ingredients

2 onions
1lb potatoes
8oz leeks, chopped
2 pints chicken stock
Mixed herbs
2oz butter
¼ pint natural yoghurt

Method

Chop onions roughly. Peel potatoes and cut into small chunks. Cut leeks into segments.

Melt the butter in a large pan and sauté the onions and potatoes for a few minutes. Add the stock, herbs and leeks. Simmer until potatoes are cooked. Allow to cool for ten minutes.

Mix in the yoghurt, then put the soup through a blender at maximum speed.

Serve hot or cold.

CLIFF RICHARD

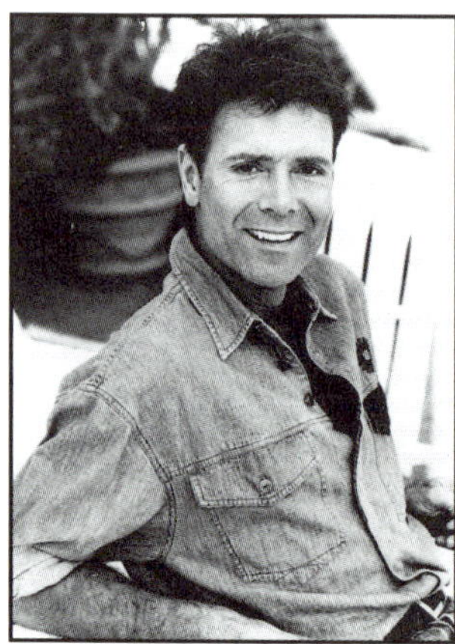

Grant's Chicken Salad Soup

Ingredients

A chicken carcass
A large onion
Garlic, if you like
2 lettuces
Any other green salad: watercress (brilliant), spring onions, chicory, cress, parsley, you name it.

The usual:
flour, butter, milk, pepper and salt. Don't ask me about quantities. You will have more idea than me.

Method

Ignoring the shallow ingratiation of the cat, dismember the chicken with your bare, cleanish hands. Put all the bits which look edible onto a plate. Place plate well out of cat's reach. Relent momentarily, and toss the cat a small piece of leg meat. Revel in your magnanimity. That's what pets are for.

Chuck all the inedible bits of chicken into a large saucepan of water, and boil furiously for half an hour or so. (Keep topping up the water.) Meanwhile shred the lettuce and other greenery, chop up the onion, crush the garlic, and cram the lot into the large frying pan in which you have just melted slightly more butter than you thought you needed. Put a lid on that, and cook it really slowly for 10 or 15 minutes, turning the resultant mess occasionally in a professional manner.

When the greenery has wilted beyond repair, scoop it all into the liquidiser, together with a cupful of the chicken stock. Scrunge it mercilessly, put it into another saucepan (it's a real kitchen-wrecker, this recipe) and add the sieved chicken stock, which should be about ready by now. Throw in what's left of the chicken meat after the cat found it after all.

Heat it all up and taste it. Delicious, eh? Alright, put the salt and pepper in then.

continued

Grant's Chicken Salad Soup (cont.)

Method (cont.)

Now make a white sauce, and bung that in as well. Cook it all up for a bit.

If you're feeling posh, you will have sliced some bread, brushed it with olive oil and garlic, sprinkled it generously with grated cheese and left it in a hot oven for 15 minutes.

Having ladled out the soup, sprinkle it with parsley and cress, and float one of the *croutes* on each dish. *Très Français, quoi?*

Serve, and deal modestly with the inevitable applause.

Comments

A spectacularly delicious yet wholly idiot-proof way of dealing with a Sunday chicken carcass and the bits of greenery which you keep meaning to throw out of the fridge.

GRANT BAYNHAM
of BBC's "That's Life"

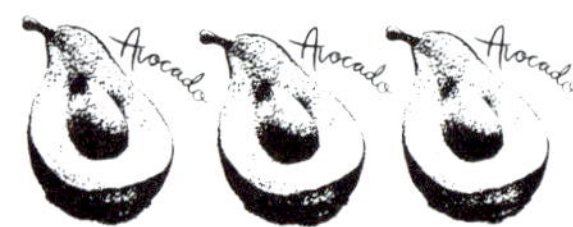

Chilled Prawn Soup

Ingredients

1 large can evaporated milk (chilled)
4 tablespoons lemon juice
2 teaspoons finely grated onion
1 level teaspoon made mustard
2 tablespoons double cream
Salt
6oz peeled prawns, finely chopped
3 tablespoons parsley, finely chopped
Paprika

Method

Combine evaporated milk with lemon juice, onion, mustard, cream and salt to taste. Gently stir in prawns and parsley. Pour into glasses/soup cups, sprinkle tops lightly with paprika and chill for at least an hour before serving.

Serve with toast.

M. JENKINS
Southwark Branch

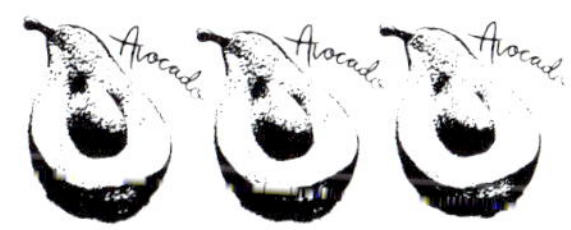

Camembert Soup

Ingredients

1 large Spanish onion, chopped
½oz butter
2 tablespoons plain flour
¾ pint white wine
½ pint chicken stock (made with a cube)
2 small rounds of Camembert
Salt and pepper
½ pint double cream

Method

Chop the onion finely. Melt the butter in a saucepan and add the onion. Cook for 5-10 minutes. Add the flour and cook for another 5 minutes. Pour the wine and stock into the pan, bring to the boil and simmer for 20 minutes.

Meanwhile, cut the rind off the Camembert and cut the cheese into cubes. Add the cheese to the soup, cook for another 10 minutes. Do not boil. Just slightly simmer or the soup will curdle. (Up to this point you can do the day before.) Add the double cream and season well to taste.

Serves 4-6.

SUSANNAH GOOCH

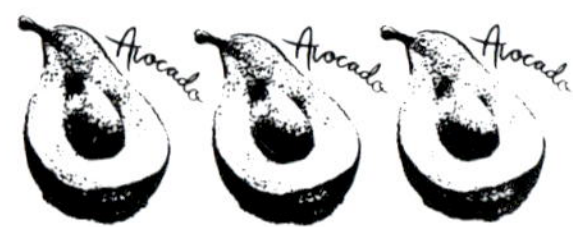

Carrot and Apple Soup

Ingredients

1 onion peeled
1lb carrots peeled
8oz cooking apples, peeled and cored
1½oz butter
1½ pints chicken stock (made with 1 stock cube)
Seasoning
Chives (optional)

For croutons:
2 slices wholemeal bread
2 tablespoons sunflower or soya oil

Method

Chop onion, carrots and apples into 1 inch cubes. Melt butter in large saucepan. Add onion, carrots and apples and cook for 5 minutes, stirring occasionally. Season generously and add 1½ pints of chicken stock. Bring to the boil. Simmer for 15 minutes.

Make up the croutons. Cut the bread into ½ inch cubes and fry in the oil until pale brown.

Transfer soup to food processor or to a blender and blend. Sprinkle the croutons on the soup just before serving. Sprinkle with 1 tablespoon of chopped chives if liked.

Serves 4.

W. BARTLETT
Buckinghamshire Branch

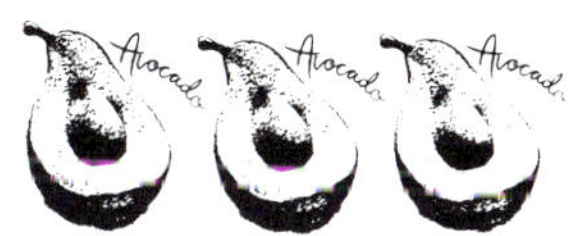

Cream of Corn Soup

Ingredients

1 tin creamed corn
Small onion
1 bay leaf
¾ pint water
1oz margarine
1 tablespoon flour
¾ pint milk
1 chicken cube
Seasoning

Method

Put corn, chopped onion, bay leaf, stock cube and water into pan. Simmer for 10 minutes.

Melt margarine over low heat. Stir in flour. Add milk slowly, stirring all the time. When the sauce thickens, add it to the corn mixture.

Season to taste with plenty of pepper and a little sugar.

THELMA LOODMER

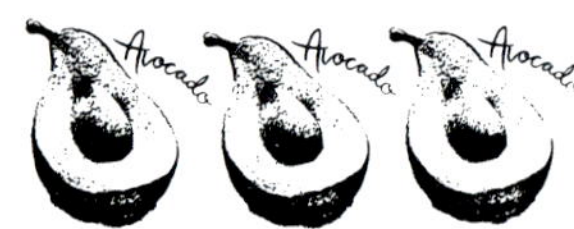

Portuguese Green Soup

Ingredients

2 pints potato water
1 pint milk
1 finely chopped cooked onion
3 medium-sized cooked sieved potatoes
3 teacups chopped cooked cabbage
Sprinkle of nutmeg

Method

Heat milk and potato water together. Add sieved potato, chopped onion and cabbage. Add seasoning. Boil fast for 3 minutes.

Serve hot.

VEENA JACKSON
Nottingham Branch

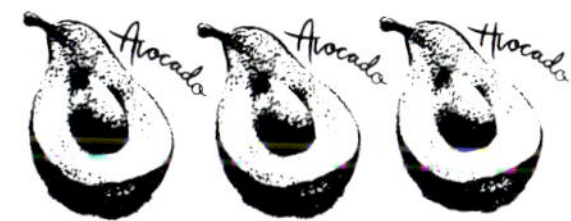

Celeriac Soup with Dill

Ingredients

8oz celeriac
4oz onion
1oz butter
1¼ pints light stock
Salt and pepper
2 tablespoons single cream
Lemon juice
Pinch of diced dill

Method

Peel and slice celeriac and onion. Melt butter and sauté gently in butter for 1 to 2 minutes. Cover with damp greaseproof paper and tight fitting lid. Cook gently for 10 minutes. Pour on stock and seasoning, bring to the boil and simmer for 30 minutes. Cool and blend (can be frozen at this stage). Return to pan and reheat. Away from heat, stir in cream, dash of lemon juice and dill. Season to taste.

Comments

Recently a friendly neighbour in our Norfolk village, who often leaves vegetables from his kitchen garden at our front door, produced a vegetable which I in my 'town-born' ignorance had never heard of – a celeriac. What is more the next day he brought round a recipe which I know he won't mind me telling you about in such a good cause. I greeted it with acclamation as I have in recent years become a soup enthusiast. This one is delicious and don't worry too much if you haven't any dill – it is still very good without it.

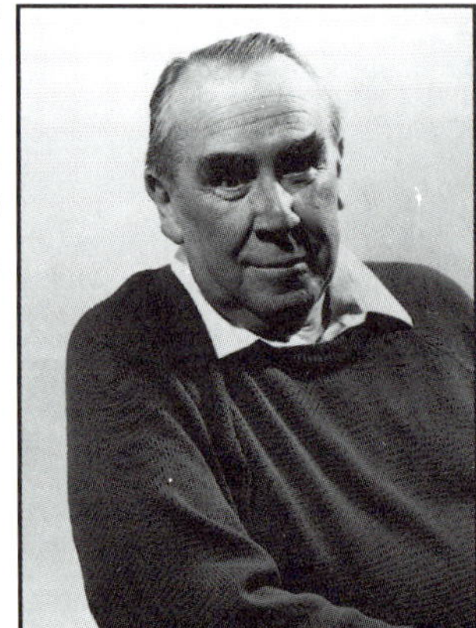

However, I can't resist the temptation to sing:

"Dill, dill, glorious dill.
You can drink pints and it won't make you ill.
So follow me follow down to the hollow,
Where celeriacs wallow with glorious dill."

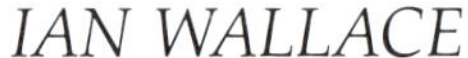

IAN WALLACE

Gower Oyster Soup

SWP WYSTRYS BRO GWYR

Ingredients

2lbs scrag end of mutton
2oz pearl barley
1 medium-sized onion
1 medium-sized turnip
Salt and black pepper
Pinch of mace
2oz butter
1½oz flour
4 dozen bearded oysters

Method

Wash meat and cut off excess fat. Place in a saucepan, add 3 pints of water. Bring to the boil, skim off any fat on surface of liquid. Wash barley, peel and dice vegetables. Add all to the pan, season to taste. Cover and simmer for 1½-3 hours.

Melt butter in pan, add flour and mix. Pour in the mutton broth stirring all the time. Simmer for 10 minutes.

Serve with the oysters lying on the bottom of their opened shells.

Serves 4-6.

NEATH AND PORT TALBOT BRANCH

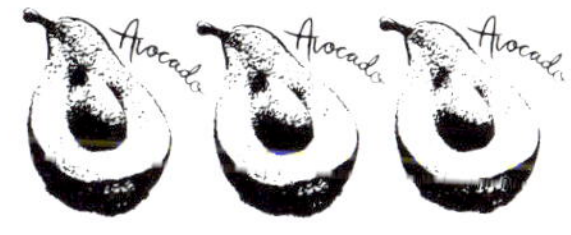

Archers Soup

Method

Put the kettle on.

Sauté half an onion in a lump of butter.

Chop up some scrubbed carrots, swedes, turnips, potatoes, celery.

Add them to the onion.

Bung in a lump of Vecon.

Top up with boiling water: add salt, pepper, savory and thyme.

Simmer.

Blend a bit of it.

Mix it all up.

Put on the "Archers".

Have it.

Best wishes,

VICTORIA WOOD

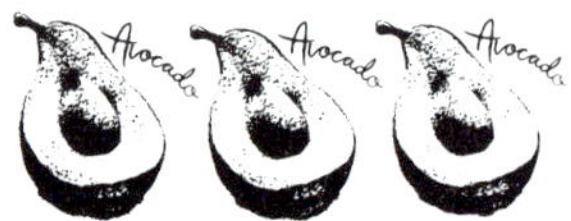

Pilchard Paté

Ingredients

Large tin of pilchards in tomato sauce (16oz)
2-3oz butter or margarine
2-3oz plain flour
½ pint milk
Salt and pepper
1 tablespoon lemon juice

Method

Make a white sauce with the flour, fat and milk by melting the fat, adding the flour and stirring over heat to make a roux. Add the milk, salt and pepper and bring to the boil, stirring. Cook till smooth. Remove from heat. Mash the pilchards, taking out the skin and bones if you prefer. To the white sauce, add the pilchards and lemon juice. Mix well: it can be put in a liquidiser to make it really smooth but this is not essential.

Transfer into several small pots or containers. As it is, it will keep in the fridge for three days. Any surplus (and it does make quite a lot) can be frozen for future use.

For decoration, lemon slices and watercress can be put on top, but it gets eaten so quickly, this hardly seems worth the effort. Serve with toast.

AUDREY FRANKLIN
Newbury and District Support Group

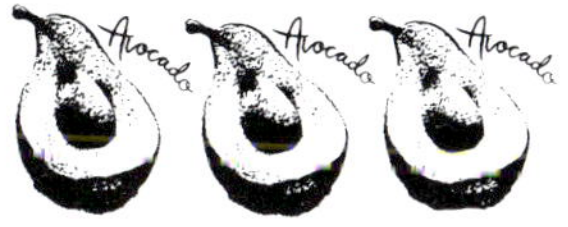

Hilary's Grandmother's Recipe for Chopped Liver

Ingredients

2lbs chicken liver (calves liver may be used)
1 large Spanish onion
3-4 hard-boiled eggs
1 teaspoon melted chicken fat (optional)
Oil for frying onions and liver
Salt and pepper to taste

Method

Fry the sliced onion in a little oil until golden for about 10 minutes. Remove from the pan. Chop in food processor for about 1 minute until very finely chopped. Place in a bowl. Fry the livers for about 10 minutes until well done. Chop in food processor until smooth. Add to the onions. Reserving one egg yolk for garnishing, finely chop hard-boiled eggs in food processor. Add to liver and onions and mix to a smooth paste. If it is not moist enough a little of the pan juices may be added or about one tablespoon of chicken fat. Season to taste with salt and pepper.

Garnish with chopped egg yolk.

Comments

I learnt this recipe from Hilary's grandmother, which is why it is named after her. Hilary is married to our "That's Life" producer, Richard Woolf.

ESTHER RANTZEN

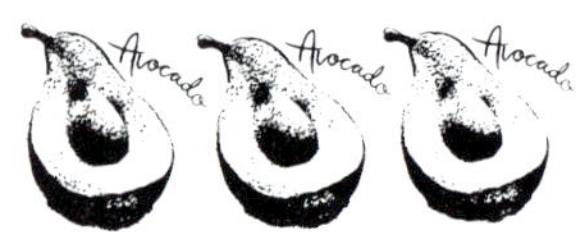

Summer Soup

Ingredients

1 can of cream of celery soup
An equal amount of tomato juice, then a dash more!
Juice of half a lemon
Pinch of cayenne pepper
Prawns
Cream
Parsley

Method

Whisk soup and juice together until smooth. Season to taste. Then add lots of luscious prawns, swirl in some cream and finish with chopped parsley. Serve chilled.

JAN HARVEY
of "Howard's Way"

Quick Pea Soup

Ingredients

1lb frozen peas
1 medium-sized onion, chopped
Salt and pepper
1½ pints chicken stock

Method

Put all ingredients in saucepan. Boil for 10 minutes. Put in liquidiser and reheat. Serve with croutons.

MYRA JANNON

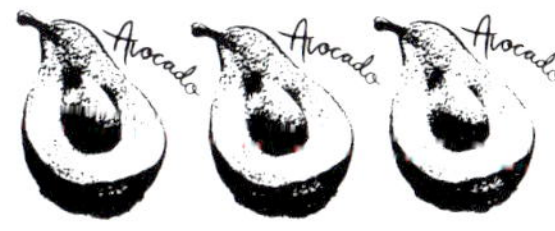

Cheesy Avocados with Prawns

Ingredients

2 avocados
8oz prawns
4 crabsticks
½ pint cheese sauce
Grated cheese

Method

Skin and halve pears and place in oven-proof dish. Cover with prawns and chopped crabsticks. Pour over cheese sauce, sprinkle with grated cheese. Put in moderate oven 10-15 minutes or until heated through.

Two avocados make a starter for 4 people or main meal with garnish and French bread for 2 people.

COLCHESTER STANWAY TOWNSWOMEN'S GUILD

Cashew Nutters

Ingredients

4oz soft margarine
2oz semolina
3½oz self-raising flour
3oz grated cheese
Salt, ground black pepper
½ teaspoon dry mustard
Cashew nuts

Method

Mix together all the ingredients except nuts and then roll into approximately 40 small balls. Place on large greased baking sheet. Press nuts, halved, on top of balls – not too deeply as they will disappear. Bake in oven at 180°C/350°F (gas mark 4) for 15-20 minutes.

KATHRYN ROBINSON

Fish Dishes

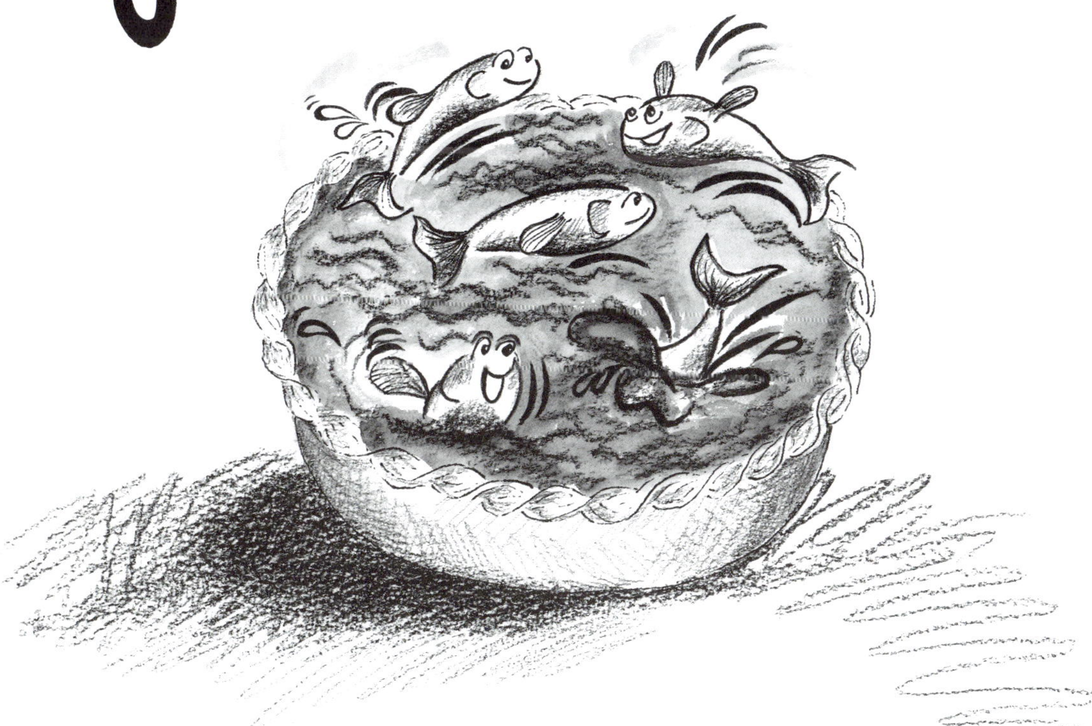

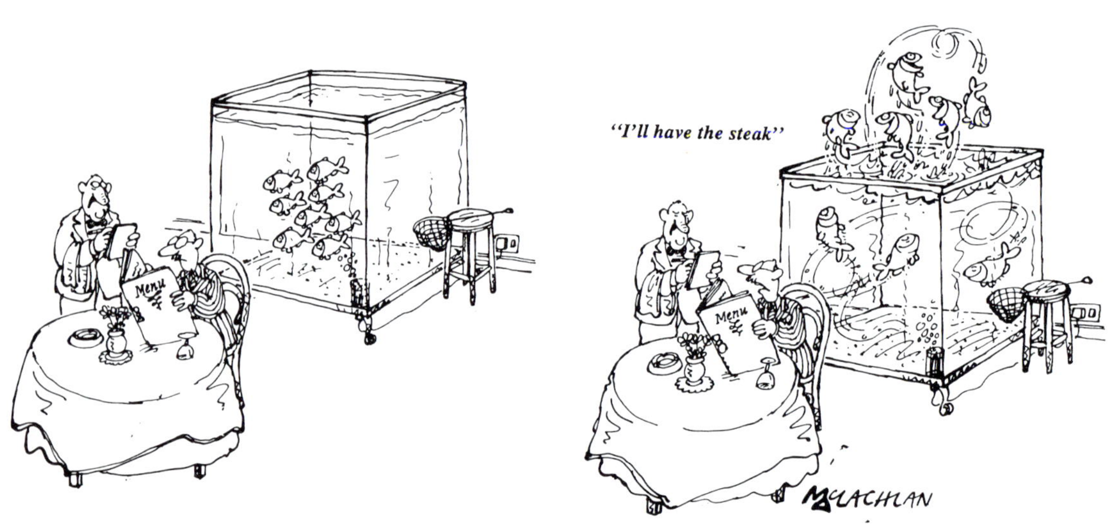

Cartoon courtesy of Ian Hislop, *Private Eye*

Macaroni and Tuna Pie

Ingredients

6oz macaroni
8oz can tuna

3 tomatoes
2 hard-boiled eggs

For cheese sauce:
1½oz butter
6 tablespoons plain flour
1 pint milk

3 oz grated cheddar cheese
Salt and pepper

Method

Cook the pasta for about 12 minutes in boiling salted water until tender. Shell and chop the eggs. Slice the tomatoes. Melt the butter in a saucepan, add flour and gradually beat in the milk. Bring to the boil and cook for about 3 minutes. Stir in 2oz of the cheese and the pasta and season with salt and pepper.

Layer the ingredients in a pie dish, finishing with a layer of the sauce. Sprinkle the other 1oz of cheese on the top. Bake at about 180°C/350°F (gas mark 4) for 30 minutes.

Garnish with a little sliced tomato and sprigs of parsley, and serve hot.

JAMES HERRIOTT

Comments

James Herriott's wife says he is a great pasta fan and this is one of his favourites.

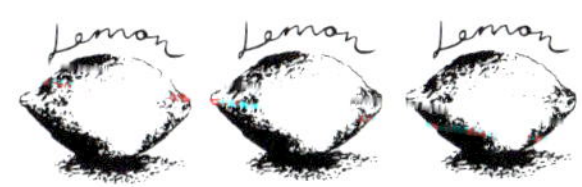

La Crème De La Crème De La Scampi

Ingredients

1½lbs frozen scampi (thawed)
Seasoned flour
2oz butter
4oz perfect button mushrooms (sliced)
1 glass of brandy
1 small carton double cream
Few sprigs of chopped parsley

Method

Dip the scampi in seasoned flour. Heat the butter. Gently fry the scampi for about 10 minutes. (You can use oil instead of butter if you'd rather.) Add the mushrooms and the brandy and cook for about another 15 minutes then add the cream. Cook until it's heated through but not boiling.

Sprinkle with parsley before serving with plain, boiled rice.

Comments

As a vegetarian from birth, I'm always on the look out for anything fishy. How about this?

DON MACLEAN

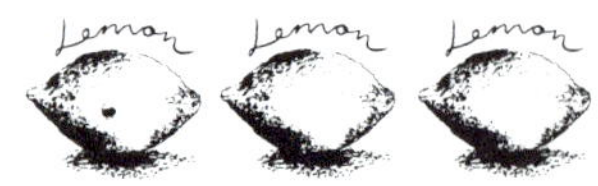

Cod & Spinach Oregano

Ingredients

4 cod fillets
Broccoli
Spinach

Paprika
1 tablespoon margarine, melted
Salt and pepper to taste

For sauce:
12oz skimmed milk
1½oz bread, crumbed
3oz grated Parmesan cheese

½ teaspoon oregano
1 teaspoon chicken stock powder

Method

Season fish with salt and pepper. Par boil vegetables and put in the bottom of baking dish. Place fish and margarine on top, sprinkle with paprika and bake in a moderate oven for 20 minutes.

For sauce:
Combine ingredients in saucepan, simmer for 5 minutes. Pour onto the fish.

Serve hot with pasta or baby new potatoes.

NERYS HUGHES

Bon appetit!
love
Nerys Hughes

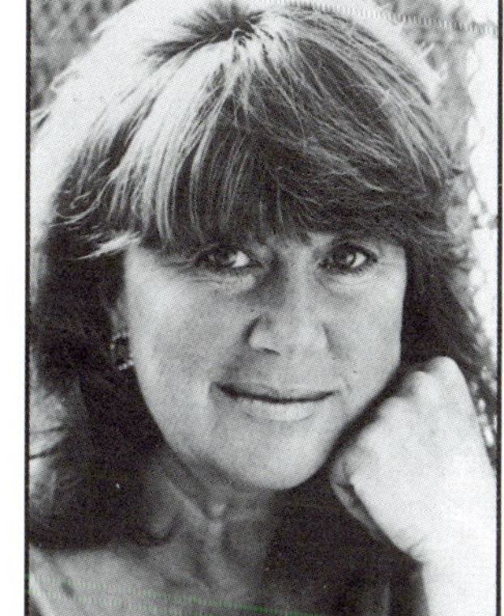

Prawn and Cheese Quiche

Ingredients

For pastry:
6 oz flour, preferably plain
Pinch salt
3oz margarine, butter or cooking fat
Water to mix

For filling:
2 eggs
¼ pint milk
Seasoning
4oz Cheddar or Lancashire cheese
4oz shelled, cooked prawns, chopped

For garnish:
Few whole prawns and parsley

Method

Sieve the flour and salt, rub in the fat, then add sufficient water to make a firm pastry of rolling consistency. Roll, cut and line a shallow 8″ flan ring or sandwich tin, or oven-proof baking dish. Bake blind for 15 minutes in the centre of hot oven at 220°C/425°F (gas mark 7). Meanwhile, beat the eggs with the seasoning. Add the warmed milk, cheese and prawns. Pour into baked pastry, return to the oven and continue baking in a moderate oven at 180°-190°/350°-375°F (gas mark 4-5) for about 25-30 minutes until the filling is firm.

Garnish with the prawns and parsley. You can serve hot or cold.

PEGGY HAMPSON
Yeovil Branch

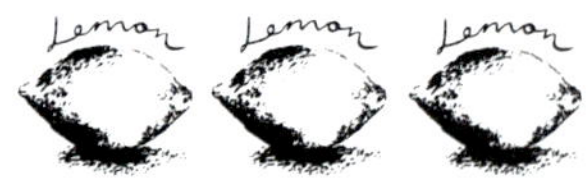

Fish Canelloni

Ingredients

For filling:

Two 7oz tins middle cut salmon
2 tablespoons mayonnaise
2 chopped hard-boiled eggs
Salt, pepper and Tabasco to taste
½ teaspoon chopped pickled cucumber
2 teaspoons sandwich spread

For crêpes:

1½ cups flour
2 cups water
½ teaspoon black pepper
Pinch of salt
3 eggs

To finish:

½ pint sour cream
4oz cheddar cheese

Method

For filling:

Remove bone from fish and flake. Mix together all ingredients and blend with fish.

For crêpes:

Add water to eggs and beat well. Add sifted flour and salt and black pepper. Grease small frying pan lightly with flour and heat. Pour batter to form thin coat on bottom of pan and cook till dry, then invert pan onto absorbent paper. Place a spoonful of fish mixture on each crêpe. Roll up, tucking in ends and place in a greased oven-proof dish. Pour over ½ pint sour cream and sprinkle with grated cheddar cheese. Bake in a moderate oven for 30 minutes.

PAULA DAWE
National Appeals Officer

Russian Fish Pie

Ingredients

8oz white fish
¼ pint milk
¼ pint water
8oz frozen flakey pastry – any pastry will be alright
½oz butter
½oz flour
3oz grated cheese
1 dessertspoon chopped parsley
Salt and pepper
Beaten egg to glaze

Method

Wash the fish and poach gently in the milk and water until cooked. Meanwhile roll pastry to a 9″ square and place on baking tray. Drain the fish reserving ¼ pint of the liquid. Skin, bone and flake the fish.

Melt butter, add flour, and stir in liquid gradually. Bring to boil and cook for 2-3 minutes. Add fish, cheese and parsley. Season with salt and pepper.

Pile mixture into the centre of the pastry square. Moisten edges, fold each corner to centre, forming an envelope. Seal leaving a small central incision for the escape of steam. Brush with egg and bake in a moderate oven for 30-35 minutes until golden.

SIR JAMES ANDERTON
Chief Constable of Greater Manchester

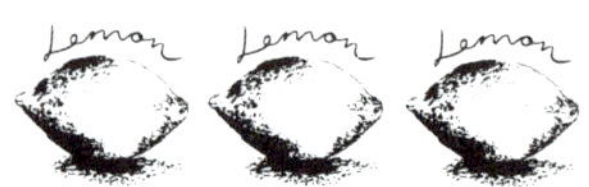

Ragout of Fresh Scallops

Ingredients

20 fresh scallops
2 medium carrots
2 medium courgettes
1 turnip
2oz wild rice
1oz finely chopped shallots
1 clove crushed garlic
1oz unsalted butter
1oz chopped chives
3 fl oz Pernod
3 fl oz white wine
½ pint fish stock
Pinch of saffron
Fennel to garnish
Salt and freshly ground white pepper

Method

Soak the wild rice in cold water for 10 minutes, then drain. Place the rice in a saucepan, add ¼ pint of fish stock and season. Bring to the boil and simmer for 20 minutes until cooked. Keep hot. Turn carrots, courgettes and turnip into small barrel shapes about 1″ long by ½″ wide.

Blanch the shallots in butter without colouring, add the white wine, Pernod and fish stock and bring to simmering point. Add the cleaned scallops and gently poach for 3 minutes. When cooked, take from cooking liquour and keep warm. Reduce stock by two-thirds and add cream and saffron. When thickened add cooked scallops and chopped chives. Arrange a timbale of wild rice on the plate then add the ragout of scallops. Garnish with turned vegetables, boiled in seasoned salted water to taste, and sprigs of fennel. Serves 4.

THOMAS GORDON
Master Builders Hotel, Buckler's Hard, Nr Beaulieu in Hampshire

Submitted by
PAT FARQUHARSON
Southport and Formby Support Group

Spinach with Shrimps or Prawns

Ingredients

1-2lbs fresh shrimps or prawns
2lbs fresh spinach
1 medium onion
4 fresh tomatoes
1 tablespoon tomato paste
1 Maggi cube
½ teaspoon black or white pepper
1 teaspoon hot pepper sauce
3 tablespoons vegetable oil

Method

Pick and wash the spinach in lukewarm water. Drain in a strainer. Cut the spinach into large strips and set aside. Boil the water in a saucepan, add 1 tablespoon of salt then blanch the spinach for about 2 minutes and strain.

Blend the fresh tomatoes and onions in the blender. Place a pot on the fire; when it is hot pour in the vegetable oil. Cook the tomato and onion mixture in the oil for about 10 minutes, add the tomato paste and cook for further 8-12 minutes stirring all the time. Add ½ cup of water and the seasonings to taste. When the vegetable is ready to serve, add the fresh shrimps and cook for only 3 minutes. Add the spinach. Serve hot.

MRS BUNMI ANYAOKU
Wife of the Commonwealth Secretary General, Chief Emeke Anyaoku

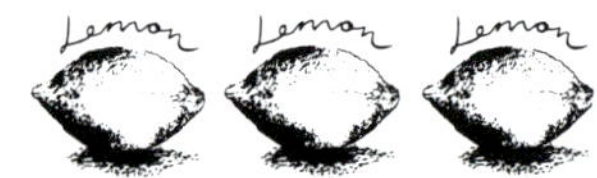

Cleo's Fish Stew

Ingredients

½ pint water
¼ cup wine vinegar or lemon juice
1 small onion sliced
1 stalk celery sliced
1 medium carrot sliced (and any other vegetable to be used up)
Fish or vegetable stock cube
Salt and pepper
1 bay leaf, pinch of thyme (or herbs to taste)
3 or 4 sprigs of parsley, if possible
8-12oz white fish pieces (skinned and boned)
A few prawns, crab sticks, mussels or any seafood

Method

Combine all ingredients except fish. Bring to boil, then reduce heat and simmer for at least 30 minutes. Add white fish, stir and cook until fish is tender.

Add seafood and cook for a few minutes. Use a small amount of cornflour to thicken if required. Serve.

Comments

Ask for leftover fish from the fishmonger. He will bone and skin it which makes the ingredients relatively inexpensive. Leftover vegetables can also be put in. Make double and freeze half. For a special occasion, add dry white wine and a little cream.

CLEO LAINE

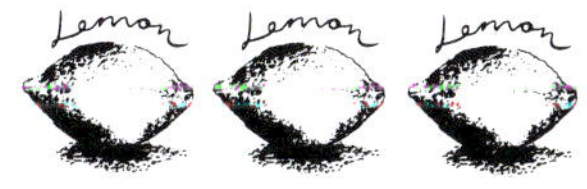

Salmon Puffs

Ingredients

1½lbs cooked salmon
½ onion
2 cloves garlic or less
7oz cream cheese
Small double cream
4oz mushrooms
6 large vol-au-vent cases, frozen
6 prawns to decorate and watercress

Method

Skin, bone and flake salmon into chunks. Very finely chop onion, mushrooms and garlic and 'sweat' in butter till soft but not brown. Beat together cheese and cream and fold in salmon and mushroom mix. Cook vol-au-vent cases following instructions. Fill with mixture on baking tray. Bake for 20 minutes approx at 180°C/350°F (gas mark 4). Garnish with prawns and watercress and serve hot.

Serves 6.

Comments

Special meal – loads of cholesterol!

Inexpensive!

Can be prepared the night before.

DEBI JONES
Daytime UK TV and Radio Merseyside

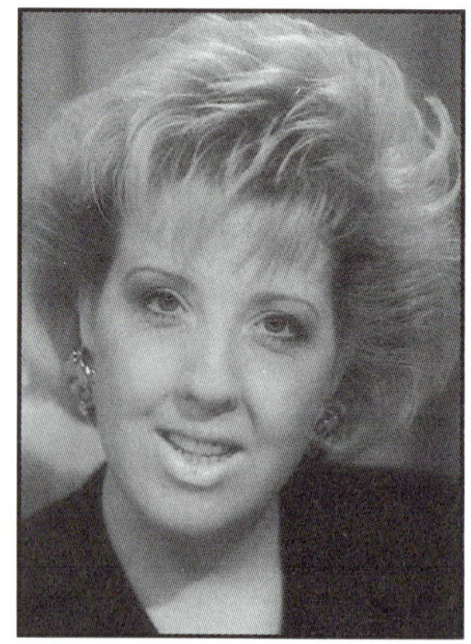

Salmon en Croute

Ingredients

4 8oz salmon fillets, skinned
4 leaves spinach
1 onion, sliced
1 bay leaf
4-5 whole peppercorns
Parsley
Fresh fennel

Equal quantities: white wine, wine vinegar and water – enough to barely cover fish
1 egg beaten
Salt and freshly ground black-pepper
16 sheets filo pastry

For sauce:
Fish stock
1oz butter
1oz flour
2 tablespoons fresh fennel

Method

Poach salmon in white wine, wine vinegar and water, with onion, bay leaf, peppercorns and salt until three-quarters cooked. Remove salmon and leave to cool. Save stock. Blanch spinach leaves and drain. Leave to cool flat. Then wrap each salmon fillet in a spinach leaf. Preparc filo pastry and wrap each parcel in 4 sheets of pastry – one at a time, brushing each one with beaten egg. Place on a greased tray and bake for 20 minutes 180°C/350°F (gas mark 4) until brown and crisp.
For sauce:
Strain stock from poaching. Melt the butter in saucepan and add flour. Cook until crumbly. Remove from heat and add the stock gradually. Return to heat, stirring until the sauce is smooth and coats the spoon. Add seasoning to taste and 2 or more tablespoons chopped fresh fennel. Decorate with sprigs of fresh fennel or parsley.

Serves 4.

ANDREW WHEATCROFT
Chef, Lloyds Bistro, Coldharbour, Dorset

Submitted by
COLIN KILBY, Yeovil, Sherborne and District Branch

Caramel Crispy Fish

Ingredients

1 tin tuna
2oz prawns
1 tin condensed mushroom or chicken soup
2oz bread
2oz cheese
1 packet prawn cocktail crisps
Lemon and parsley to garnish

Method

Heat the oven to 190°C/375°F (gas mark 5).

Place fish and prawns in greased oven-proof dish, pour soup over fish. Grate cheese and bread, crush crisps and mix together. Place over soup. Bake in centre of oven for 30 minutes until lightly browned.

Garnish with lemon and parsley and serve.

VINCENT BILLINGTON
International concert pianist, Scarborough

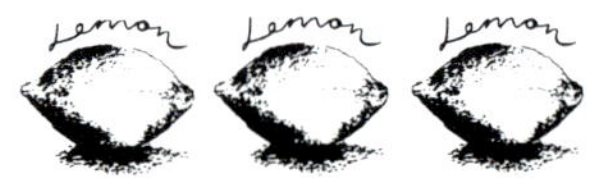

Doyle's Stuffed King Prawns

Ingredients

24 large, uncooked prawns

Oil, for frying

For filling:
1 onion, finely chopped
1 clove garlic, crushed
1 tablespoon butter
4 slices thick bacon, rinded and finely chopped
4oz frozen, chopped spinach, thawed and drained
1 large egg
2 tablespoons chopped, fresh parsley
2 tablespoons fresh breadcrumbs
Pinch of salt
3oz sultanas, soaked in wine and drained

For batter:
10oz plain flour
12fl oz can lager
1 teaspoon salt
2 egg whites

For sauce:
1 small jar fruit chutney
1 tablespoon curry powder
6 shallots, chopped
1 small jar mayonnaise

Method

First make the filling. Lightly fry the onion and garlic in butter. Add the remainder of the filling ingredients, using enough of the fresh breadcrumbs to bind the mixture. Set aside.

Then make the batter. Put the flour in a deep bowl and slowly add the lager. Add the salt and mix to a smooth, thin batter. Lightly beat the egg whites and if necessary add a little extra flour. The batter should be thin but with body.

continued

Doyle's Stuffed King Prawns (cont.)

Method (cont.)

Butterfly the prawns by cutting each down to the start of the tail and gently flatten the sides. De-vein and de-head. Fill the cut section of the butterfly prawns with the filling mixture, pressing the sides firmly together. Chill until firm.

Prepare the sauce by carefully blending all the ingredients together. Then, when you are ready to cook, carefully dip the stuffed prawns into the batter and deep fry at 180-190°C/350-375°F (gas mark 4-5) for 5 minutes. Serve hot with the fruity sauce.

Serves 4-6.

KEITH FLOYD

Comments

This recipe will be published in the forthcoming book *Floyd on Oz*. Publisher Michael Joseph. September 1991. Mr Floyd liked this dish so much that it has been included on the menu at his pub.

Submitted by
MRS PAT BISHOP
Torquay Branch

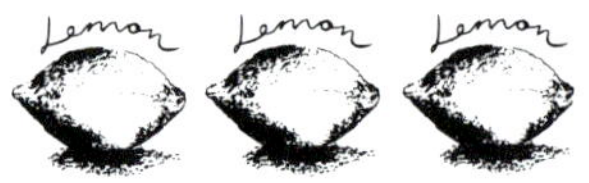

Haddock Mavroudis

Ingredients

12oz smoked haddock
1 sachet gelatine
6oz curd cheese
1 tablespoon French mustard
3 tablespoons mayonnaise
1oz chopped capers
¼ pint double cream, lightly whipped
14oz smoked salmon, thinly sliced
Lambs lettuce and lemon as garnish

Method

Poach the smoked haddock lightly till tender. Drain, reserving 3 fl. oz of cooking liquid. Sprinkle gelatine on to the reserved liquid until dissolved.

Blend together the curd cheese, mustard and mayonnaise. Flake the cooked haddock and add to this mixture, together with capers and the gelatine liquid. Add seasoning (but be careful with the salt) and fold in the whipped cream.

Line 6 ¼ pint ramikins with smoked salmon, overlapping the pieces and leaving the ends long enough to fold over the top when the ramekins are filled. Divide the haddock mix among the lined ramekins, and fold the smoked salmon over to cover it. Put clingfilm over them and refrigerate overnight.

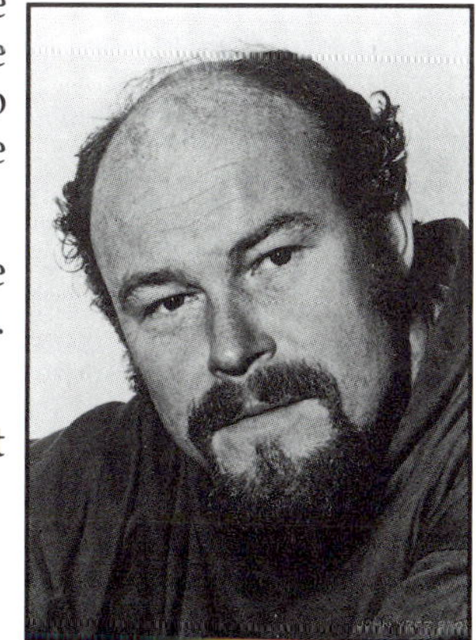

Arrange lambs lettuce on 6 plates and turn out the moulds on to the leaves. Garnish with sliced lemon. Serve with crusty bread of a serious nature.

You'll find this is almost too much for a starter – it makes a good light main dish for a summer evening.

TIMOTHY WEST

Fish Caledonia

Ingredients

1lb fish (white or smoked), cooked
1 can sweetcorn kernels
1oz margarine or butter
1oz flour
½ pint milk
Salt and pepper and pinch of mustard
2 eggs separated
2oz grated cheese

Method

Flake fish, drain sweetcorn. Melt margarine, then add flour and mix. Pour on milk and stir until simmering. Season and add mustard. Draw pan from heat and stir in corn. Beat in egg yolks and most of cheese (reserve a little for the top). Whip egg whites and fold into sauce.

Butter oven-proof dish and fill by layering fish and sauce, finishing with sauce. Sprinkle over remaining cheese and bake in moderate oven for approx 20-30 minutes.

SOUTH WEST REGIONAL OFFICE

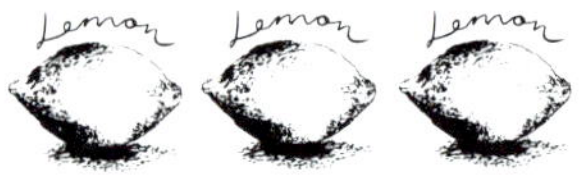

Tuna Fish Pie

Ingredients

2oz margarine
1 tablespoon flour
Enough milk to make a thick sauce
3 hard-boiled eggs
1 tin of tuna fish (with the sign that it isn't netted)
2 heads of parsley
2oz tasty cheddar cheese
Salt and freshly ground black pepper
2 sliced tomatoes (optional)
Enough mashed potato to make a 2″ cover for the above ingredients

Method

Grease a high-sided pie dish. Melt the margarine in a pan, adding the flour, salt and pepper and enough milk to make a thick white sauce. Add the grated cheese and heat until melted. To this sauce add the tin of tuna, chopped parsley and roughly chopped hard boiled eggs. Mix carefully so as not to mash the mixture and pour into your pie dish. Place the slices of tomato on top, and then the mashed potato. Dot with margarine and place in a medium to hot oven for 20-30 minutes. Serve with any vegetable.

Serves 2-3.

Comments

This is a family favourite – provided it's made with 'dolphin friendly' tuna!!

RT. HON. PADDY ASHDOWN MP

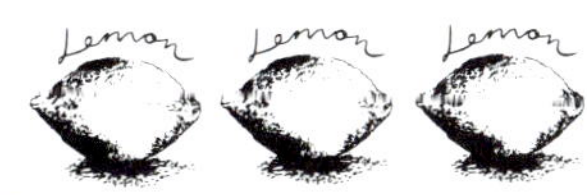

Pam's Salmon Envelope

Ingredients

1lb salmon
4 tablespoons dry white wine
Salt and freshly ground pepper
1½oz butter
1½oz plain flour
8oz hard cheese, grated
3 eggs hard boiled and roughly chopped
5fl oz soured cream

2 tablespoons chopped fresh parsley

2oz lard
1lb self-raising flour
Milk to bind
or 1lb packet of pastry

Beaten egg to glaze

Method

Place salmon in a pan of cold water, add wine and seasoning. Simmer for 20 minutes. Reserve fish stock, flake fish, discard bones and skin. Melt butter in pan, stir in flour, remove from heat and stir in ½ pint fish stock. Boil and cook for 2 minutes. Remove from heat, stir in 7oz cheese, chopped eggs, sour cream, parsley and seasoning. Cool.

Make pastry. Roll out one third of pastry into oblong. Place on well greased baking sheet. Spread sauce thickly over pastry, follow with a layer of flaked salmon, then a layer of sauce, until all salmon and sauce is used up. Cover with a lid of pastry, seal edges and decorate with pastry trimmings. Glaze and bake in oven for 40 minutes at 190°C/375°F (gas mark 5). Serve warm. Serves 6.

Comments

This is a little fiddly, but well worth it. It's very rich, and you may wish to serve it with a fishy or creamy sauce. It freezes very well!

PAM ROYLE
Tyne Tees T.V.

Submitted by
GATESHEAD BRANCH

Koulibiac

Ingredients

1lb middle cut salmon
4oz long grain rice
½ pint cold chicken stock
Salt
Freshly ground black pepper
3oz butter
4oz onions, or shallots
4oz small button mushrooms
2 tablespoons fresh chopped parsley
Juice of 1 lemon
Pinch of grated nutmeg
14oz puff pastry
2 hard-boiled eggs
1 egg beaten

To serve:
Sour cream and cucumber sauce

Method

Put the rice, stock and ¼ teaspoon salt into a saucepan and bring to the boil. Stir, cover tightly and simmer for 15-20 minutes until all the stock has been absorbed and the rice is dry and fluffy.

Cut the salmon into ¼″ slices and season with salt and pepper. Melt 2oz butter in a large frying pan and lightly fry the slices of fish for 2-3 minutes each side. Lift out and leave to cool. Peel and finely chop the onions or shallots. Add the remaining butter to the pan, put in the onion and fry gently until soft and golden. Wipe and finely slice the mushrooms. Add the mushrooms to the onions, stir well and continue frying for another 4-5 minutes.

Skin and flake the fish coarsely, carefully removing all the bones as you do so. Add the cooked rice, flaked fish and chopped parsley to the onion and

continued

Koulibiac (cont.)

Method (cont.)

mushroom mixture and season with lemon juice, nutmeg, salt and pepper to taste. Mix well and set aside to cool. Heat oven to 200°C/400°F (gas mark 6).

Divide the pastry in half and roll out each piece into an oblong measuring 12″ × 9″. Cut a 1″ strip off the shorter side of each piece and reserve. Lay one oblong of pastry on a flat baking sheet. Cover it with the cold rice and fish mixture, leaving a ½″ margin around the edges. Slice the hard-boiled eggs thinly and lay over the mixture. Dampen the edges of the pastry with water, lay the second oblong of pastry on top and press the edges together to seal them. Seal the edges with the back of a knife. Make two vent holes in the centre of the top layer of pastry for the steam to escape. Cut the reserved strips of pastry into leaves and use to decorate around the holes. Brush pastry with beaten egg. Bake towards the top of the oven for about 30-40 minutes until the pastry is cooked and golden. Serve hot with cold cucumber sauce.

Serves 8-10.

MAUREEN LIPMAN

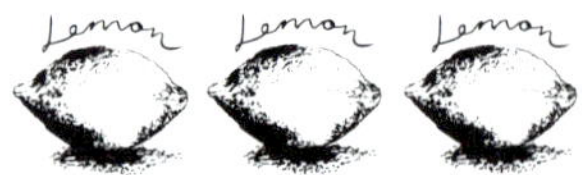

Marinated Fish Steaks

Ingredients

2 white fish steaks,
 fresh or defrosted
1 tablespoon oil
1 tablespoon Worcester sauce
1 tablespoon tomato ketchup
1 teaspoon clear honey
½ teaspoon ground ginger
½ teaspoon ground coriander
½ teaspoon paprika
½ teaspoon dry mustard
Parsley and lemon wedges
 to garnish

Method

Mix together oil, Worcester sauce, tomato ketchup, honey and dry ingredients. Spread mixture over fish steaks; cover and marinate in a cool place for 30 minutes. Shake off excess marinade and cook steaks for 8-12 minutes under a medium grill. Garnish with parsley and lemon wedges.

Serve with jacket potatoes or pasta.

EDNA CLARKE
Felixstowe Branch

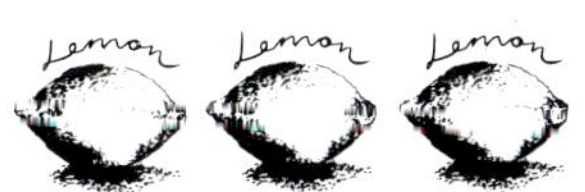

Salmon Mould

Ingredients

7½oz can red salmon
2 medium-sized eggs
1 large cup white breadcrumbs
Salt and pepper to taste

Method

Mash the salmon and breadcrumbs together. Add the salt, pepper and beaten eggs. Put into a buttered basin and steam for 1 hour. Leave to cool. When cold, turn out onto a bed of lettuce leaves and serve with other salad items.

TORBAY BRANCH

Cod with Mushrooms and Cheese

Ingredients

2 cod fillets
5-6 tablespoons mushroom soup (diluted to taste)
6 sliced button mushrooms
Frozen young sweetcorn
Grated Parmesan cheese

Method

Place fillets in a shallow oiled casserole dish. Pour over mushroom soup. Add mushrooms and sweetcorn as required. Sprinkle with cheese. Cook in a pre-heated oven 190°C/375°F (gas mark 5) for 25 minutes.

JOHN SHARMAN
Ipswich

Neopolitan Toast

Ingredients

4 large slices of bread
4oz Bel Paese cheese
4 anchovy fillets (divided down the middle to make two strips)
8 slices tomato
8 teaspoons olive oil
Oregano (dried is fine)

Method

Lay bread on oiled baking tray. Cover bread with cheese, anchovy strips and tomato slices. Sprinkle with olive oil and oregano. Bake for 15 minutes in oven at 180°C/350°F (gas mark 4).

Eat while hot – wish you'd made double.

TONY HART

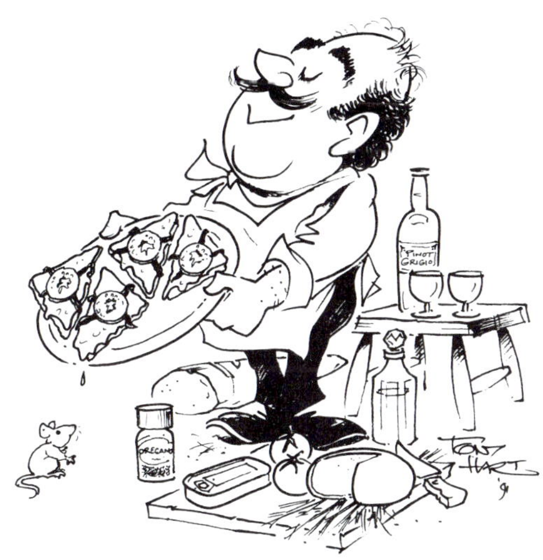

Tuna Fish Pie

Ingredients

1 tin tuna in oil
1 small cauliflower, precooked
Mashed potato, precooked
Cheese sauce
Paprika and breadcrumbs

Method

Grease an oven-proof dish. Place a layer of mashed potato on the bottom followed by the tuna, cauliflower, cheese sauce, paprika and breadcrumbs if desired. Grill or bake to taste.

M. O. PRICE
Chiswick, London

Macaroni and Tuna Bake

Ingredients

8oz short cut cooked macaroni
Salt and pepper
7oz can tuna, drained and flaked
8oz cottage cheese
3oz cheddar cheese, grated
8oz courgettes, thinly sliced
14oz can chopped tomatoes with their juice

Method

Mix all ingredients and bake at 200°C/400°F (gas mark 6) for 45 minutes or until courgettes tender.

LIVERPOOL FOOTBALL CLUB TEAM

Fried Herring

Method

Cut off heads, fins and tails of herrings required. Remove scales and wipe each fish. Score across both sides. Dry by leaving in folds of a towel for an hour or so. Sprinkle with salt and pepper and dip in coarse oatmeal until the fish are completely covered. Fry in very hot fat on both sides until a nice brown for about 6-10 minutes. Drain and serve piping hot.

RUTH FERMOY

Submitted by
MRS EMILY MILLINGTON-SMITH
Norwich Branch

Spaghetti and Tuna Dish

Ingredients

1 tin tuna fish
1 tin anchovies
Good handful parsley, chopped
4oz butter or sunflower oil
4oz packet spaghetti

Method

Open the tins of fish and mash together. While the spaghetti is cooking, melt the butter and heat the fish in it – at the last minute, sprinkle with the parsley. Drain the spaghetti. Put in a dish and toss in the fish mixture. Total time taken: 12 minutes! Serves 2-3.

MONICA UNWIN
Assistant Director (Development)

Baked Fish

Ingredients

2 large cod or haddock fillets, skinned
2 large onions sliced
2 large carrots, sliced
Salt, pepper, knobs of margarine
Milk

Method

Put all the ingredients in a casserole. Cover with milk. Bake in a slow oven for 3-4 hours.

FRANKIE VAUGHAN, OBE

Quick Pacific Pie

Ingredients

Strained tin tuna (in brine)
Tin of condensed chicken soup
2 large tomatoes, skinned
Large packet of crisps
Small packet frozen peas, cooked
Grated cheese

Method

Flake half the tuna on bottom of oven-proof pie dish. Cover with half the soup, half the peas, one sliced tomato and a layer of crisps. Repeat the process and sprinkle top with grated cheese. Place in oven gas mark 5 for 30 minutes. Brown under grill for a few minutes before serving.

EDNA DORÉ
Actress

Tuna Fish and Egg Pie

Ingredients

1 small tin tuna in oil
4 eggs
8oz cheese (grated)
½ pint white sauce
1 tomato (for garnish and colour)
½lb potatoes
Butter pat

Method

Boil potatoes and mash with butter. Hard boil eggs. Place tuna and sliced eggs in oven-proof dish. Make white sauce and add 6oz cheese. When cooked pour over eggs and tuna fish. Add mashed potato on top. Sprinkle on remaining cheese. Arrange tomato on top. Place under grill till hot. Serve with peas.

Serves 2.

Comments

Carer's note: This meal is colourful and very easy to digest and appeals readily to Alzheimer's sufferers. Preparation and cooking: 1 hour.

MRS M. A. MARFELL
Maidstone Branch

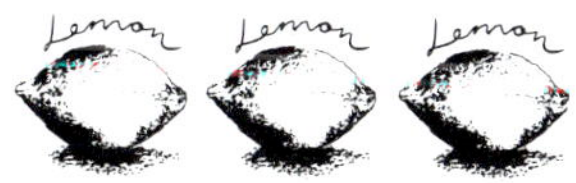

Fish Finger Sandwich

Ingredients

Fish fingers
White bread
Butter
Salt
Vinegar

Method

Cook fish fingers. Butter bread. Make sandwiches, seasoning fish fingers with salt and vinegar.

MICHAEL ELPHICK

Cold Salmon

Ingredients

Salmon

Method

Prepare fish and place in pot or fish kettle of boiling water. Allow to boil for 3 minutes. Remove from the heat and leave the fish in the water overnight. Next day you should have a perfectly cooked cold salmon.

THE RT. HON. JOHN SMITH, QC, MP

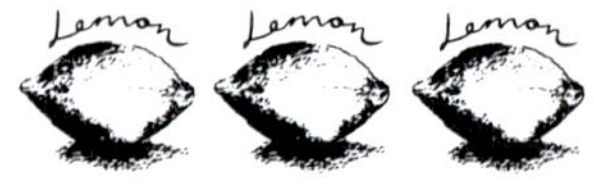

Sole Suisse

Ingredients

8 fillets sole or plaice
Juice of 1 lemon
2 10½oz cans condensed cream of mushroom soup
Salt and pepper
2 tablespoons of milk or sherry to taste
Lemon for garnish

Method

Wash and trim fillets. Sprinkle with seasoning and about half of lemon juice. Roll fish and place in greased oven-proof dish. Put soup in a basin, beat in the milk or sherry and remaining lemon juice. Pour over the fish, cover with greased paper and bake in a moderate oven for 25 minutes. Garnish with lemon

MRS B. M. PURDUE

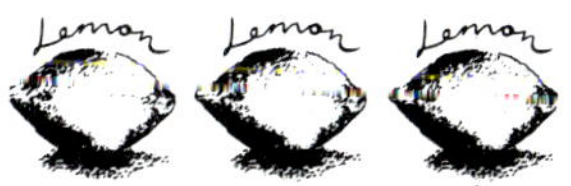

Elvers

Ingredients

1lb elvers
2 rashers of bacon
2 eggs

Method

Scald the elvers several times in salted water. Fry the rashers and put to one side. Put the elvers into the hot bacon fat, break two eggs and stir in well. Continue to cook until the elvers turn a consistent white. Dish up on rashers and serve with a dash of vinegar. If the elvers are cooked too long, the flavour is lost. Do not use very lean bacon.

Comments

When living in the Forest of Dean, Gloucester, I came across the above recipe for Elvers, a delicacy among the mining population of the Forest and purported to be an aphrodisiac!

We tried these just once because (a) I could not bear all the little eyes of the eel progeny looking at me and (b) it took ages to wash them as they were very slimy.

We moved to the Forest from the Maidstone area on my husband's retirement and had just 15 months of glorious Forest before my husband developed Alzheimer's disease. The disease progressed over 3 years when he ceased to know me. I am glad we had tasted the elvers together as it was quite an experience.

MRS E. L. MUMMERY
Maidstone Branch

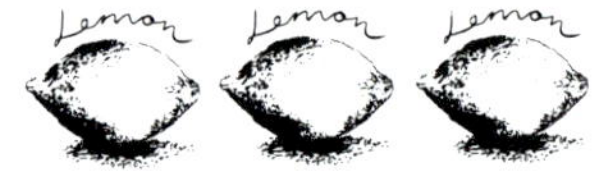

Meat & Poultry Dishes

Praise to God who giveth meat
Convenient unto all who eat
Praise for tea and buttered toast
Father, Son and Holy Ghost

Favourite Grace
Submitted by *CORA PHILLIPS*
A Founder of the Alzheimer's Disease Society

Myra's Stuffed Aubergines

Ingredients

2lbs lean minced beef
8oz chopped onions
Clove of garlic
Mixed herbs
½ pint tomato juice
Dash of Worcester sauce
3 teaspoons of Bovril
Black pepper
8 aubergines
Bread crumbs

Method

Put minced beef in a heavy-based pan, cover with water and bring to the boil for 5 minutes. Pour off the liquid, then add onions, crushed garlic, herbs and tomato juice. Mix Bovril and Worcester sauce with a little hot water and add to the mince. Simmer for 45 minutes or until tender.

Place aubergines in water and simmer until skins start to wrinkle (do not overcook!). Cut in half and scoop out flesh and mix with minced beef. Fill the aubergine shells with the mixture and bake in a moderate oven for 30 minutes. Cover with very fine bread crumbs and place under a grill to brown. Serve at once.

Serves 8.

SIR HARRY SECOMBE, CBE

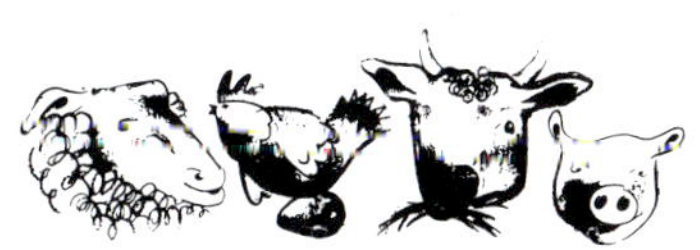

Chinese Style Steak

Ingredients

Fillet of sirloin steak
Black peppercorns
Butter
Oil
Mushrooms
Cream
Soy sauce

Method

Crush the black peppercorns in a pestle and mortar and press them into the steak. Leave for at least 20 minutes to allow the flavour to penetrate. Melt some butter in a frying pan (add a touch of oil to stop the butter burning) and add the steaks. Throw in some finely sliced mushrooms and stir them around the steak while it cooks.

When the steak is ready, add some cream and enough soy sauce to colour, until the colour and the taste are right. The sauce should be a light brown. Serve the steak with the sauce and garnish with vegetables or salad.

CILLA BLACK

Submitted by
LYNDA ROY
Hastings and Rother Branch

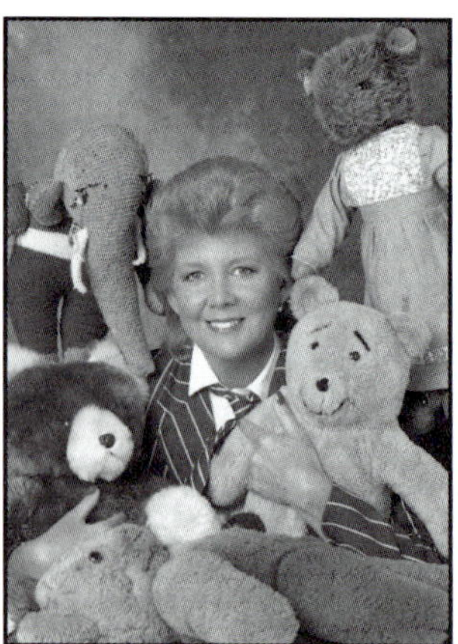

Lazy Moussaka

Ingredients

2lbs mince
8 tomatoes
2 red peppers
Mushrooms
A few aubergines
Mixed herbs
4 onions
2 green peppers
Garlic
A lot of potatoes
8oz cheese
Salt and pepper

Method

You get a big baking tin and grease it. Then you get a load of mince, onions, garlic, peppers, tomatoes, things of that nature, and fry them up in a pan. It is a good idea to do the mince first and drain off the fat. Speaking of which you could leave the mince out altogether and maybe put in mushrooms or something instead. I only say this as I am making something of an attempt to cut down on meat. This is because – let's face it – meat as food does not make a lot of environmental or economic sense in global terms and if everybody else agreed to do it I'd go veggie tomorrow. However meat is very tasty and I'm afraid this particular dish does rather need it. If you did do it without you'd probably best add a bit of stock as the mince provides some moisture.

Anyway, put in your mixed herbs or whatever and some salt and pepper and cook until it's, well, cooked. To get a bit technical the onions are best done in a separate pan and then mixed in because that way you can brown them properly. For some strange reason, known only to the creator, onions have a lot of taste when raw, then taste of absolutely nothing when cooked till white and soft, and then a lot of taste again (but completely different) when browned. Weird isn't it? Also it is nice to peel the tomatoes. This can be done by dunking them in hot

continued

Lazy Moussaka (cont.)

Method (cont.)

water, which makes the peel come off easily: why, again I do not know. The quantities required of course vary according to how much you want, but I recommend loads of everything, because it all shrinks when you cook it. For four people, at a guess I'd say four onions, eight tomatoes, two green peppers, two red, and two pounds of mince. Minimum.

Anyway, then you peel a lot of potatoes and wash a few aubergines and slice them up thinly. Having done this you put a layer of potato and aubergine slices in the bottom of the pan, then spread a layer of the mince gunk on top of that, then you put down another potato layer and then – well you get the idea. Repeat the process until you have run out of everything, being sure to finish with a good layer of spuds and aubergines. Then grate about half a pound of cheese and put that on top. Incidentally you should have heated your oven up, pretty hot – about 200°C/400°F (gas mark 6). Put the dish in the oven and give it at least an hour.

Comments

I do not often cook major meals really, but this is one which I have knocked up occasionally over the years and I must say it always goes down rather well. It is a sort of invention of my own and I call it Lazy Moussaka because it is basically moussaka without the difficult bit which is the rich creamy cheese sauce which is supposed to rise. Personally I much prefer my version which is just as well because I can't do the sauce.

BEN ELTON

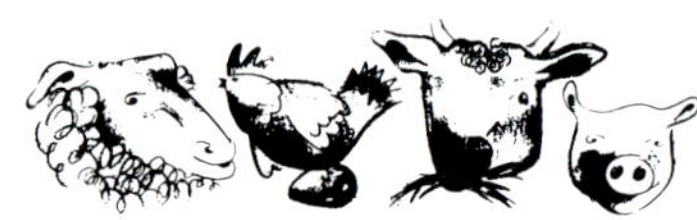

Mahone Bay Casserole

Ingredients

1 green pepper
1 large onion
8oz minced beef
Butter and oil for frying
1 can creamed corn
1 can Campbell's condensed tomato soup
Chilli powder (hot or mild)
Seasoning, bay leaf, thyme
1 can red kidney beans (optional)

Method

Sauté the pepper and onion in butter and oil. Fry the beef and drain off the fat. Mix pepper, onion, beef, soup and creamed corn with the chilli powder and seasoning to taste. A tin of red kidney beans may be added at this point. Bake for 45 minutes at 170°C/325°F (gas mark 3).

Comments

This will freeze or will keep overnight in the refrigerator.

JOAN ALCOCK

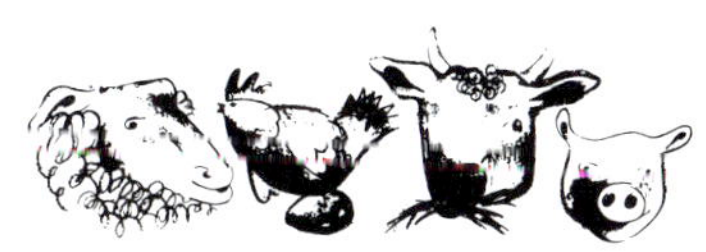

Oxtail Stew

Ingredients

1 large oxtail cut into joints, trimmed of excess fat
8oz shin of beef
2 medium onions sliced
8oz carrots, scraped and left whole
2 sticks celery, chopped
1 clove garlic, peeled and chopped
1 pint stock
½ pint red wine
1 rounded tablespoon flour
2oz beef dripping
Salt and pepper

Method

Wash the oxtail well, patting dry. Heat the dripping and fry onion and garlic for 1 minute. Add oxtail, then shin of beef and brown all over. Add carrots and celery, and cook for a further minute. Stir the flour into the juices and gradually add the stock, followed by the wine, stirring continuously. Cover and simmer very slowly for 4-5 hours until the oxtail meat is very tender and comes easily away from the bone. Alternatively, it may be braised in the oven at 150°C/300°F (gas mark 2).

Best cooked the day before you want it when any excess fat will have risen to the top and may be removed. Reheat thoroughly and season to taste.

NEWCASTLE UNITED FOOTBALL CLUB

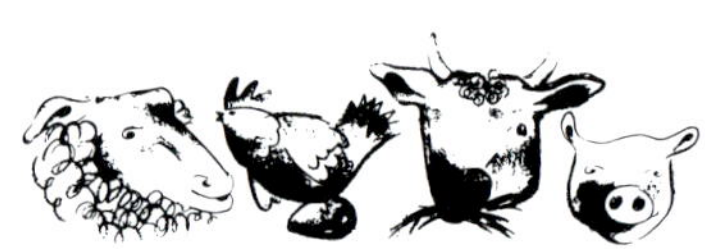

Beef Stroganoff

Ingredients

1 large onion
1lb good quality braising steak
1 tin Campbell's condensed mushroom soup undiluted
A little cream or yoghurt to add before serving
A little butter

Method

Slice the onion and brown slightly in a little butter. Remove onion from pan and add bite-sized pieces of steak to the pan and seal. Transfer both onion and sealed steak to a casserole with a tin of Campbell's condensed mushroom soup. Do not dilute the soup. Do not add salt. Leave in a low oven to bubble gently until cooked – usually about 1½-2 hours.

For a touch of the exotic add a few swirls of cream or yoghurt before serving.

Comments

This will wait ages if the eaters are late. It needs a strongly coloured vegetable as otherwise it looks rather bland.

MARY LUCAS

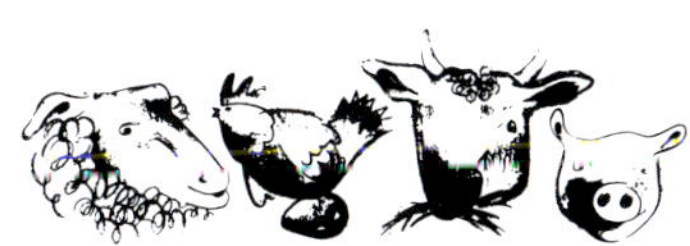

Spicy Stuffed Cabbage Leaves

Ingredients

Cooking oil
8 large cabbage leaves
1lb minced meat
Large can tomatoes
1 chopped onion
2 teaspoons cornflour
2 tablespoons Worcester sauce
Favourite herbs and seasoning
1 tablespoon chopped parsley

For sauce:
1 tablespoon tomato puree
2 teaspoons cornflour
1 teaspoon Worcester sauce
½ teaspoon sugar
Seasoning

Method

Boil cabbage leaves for 2 minutes and drain well. Heat oil in pan and fry onion until tender. Add meat and fry until browned. Drain tomatoes, keeping the juice for the sauce, and add to the meat. Blend cornflour with Worcester sauce and stir into mixture with herbs and seasoning. Cover and simmer for 20 minutes, stirring occasionally. Spoon meat stuffing onto cabbage leaves and roll up, folding over edges of leaves to enclose meat completely. Place in greased shallow dish, cover and cook in oven at 180°C/350°F (gas mark 4) for 20 minutes.

For sauce:
Blend juice from canned tomatoes with tomato puree and make up to ½ pint with water. Blend cornflour with 1 tablespoon of this tomato juice. Put all sauce ingredients in pan, bring to the boil and stir. Reduce heat and cook gently for 3 minutes. Season to taste. Pour sauce over cabbage leaves.

Serve with baked jacket potatoes and salad.

POLLY HEMMINGWAY and ROY MARSDEN

Yorkshireman's Goose

Ingredients

8oz ox liver
1 onion
1lb potatoes
1 teaspoon flour
½ teaspoon pounded sage
Stock or water
Salt and pepper

Method

Wash, wipe and slice liver. Put the flour on a plate, season liver with salt and pepper and dip it in the flour. Place the slices in layers in a greased dish.

Parboil the onion, mince it, mix it with the sage, and sprinkle between the layers of liver, pouring in sufficient stock (or water) to come half way up the dish. Parboil the potatoes, cut them in slices, place them over the top of liver to form a crust. Bake for an hour until the top potatoes are nicely browned.

J. BOWKER
York Branch

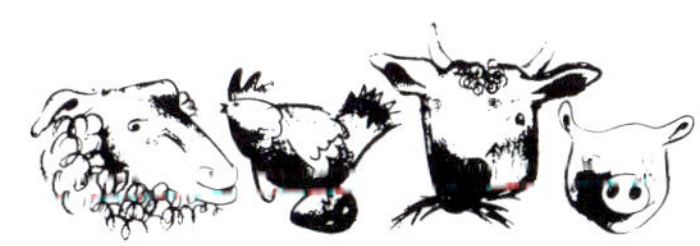

Beef in Stout

Ingredients

1½oz butter
1 tablespoon vegetable oil
2lbs stewing steak, cut into 2 inch cubes
4 medium-sized onions, skinned and sliced
8oz button mushrooms, halved
Salt and pepper
2 tablespoons plain flour
½ pint stout
1 bayleaf
1 teaspoon soft dark brown sugar

Method

Heat the butter and oil in a large flame-proof casserole and cook the meat for 10 minutes, until brown all over. Remove the meat from the pan with a slotted spoon. Add the onions and mushrooms to the pan, adding more oil if necessary, and fry until softened. Season to taste, add the flour and stir well so that the flour absorbs the fat.

Return the meat to the pan, pour in the stout and add the bay leaf and brown sugar. Stir well, mix. Cover and cook gently, either on top of the stove or in the oven at 180°C/350°F (gas mark 4) for about 2½ hours or until the meat is tender.

Serves 4-6.

CLIVE HORNBY
Jack Sugden in 'Emmerdale Farm'

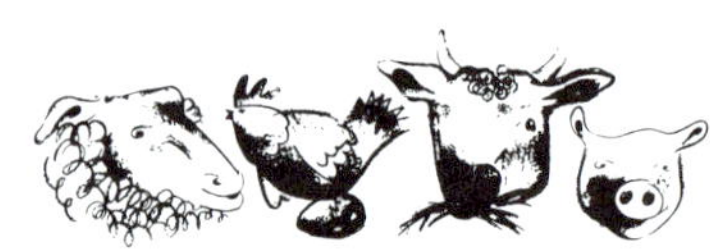

Chilli Con Carne

Ingredients

1lb minced beef
1 large can plum tomatoes
1 large can kidney beans
1 large can baked beans
¼ pint beef stock
Dash Worcester sauce
1 clove garlic
2 medium-sized onions
2 tablespoons tomato puree
1 tablespoon olive oil
Salt and freshly ground pepper
1½ teaspoon hot chilli powder
1 teaspoon mixed herbs
1 bayleaf

Method

Slice onion, season with pepper and crushed garlic. Fry in olive oil till soft. Add mince, fry until well-browned. Add drained kidney beans, beef stock and bay leaf. Stir and add tomato puree and tomatoes. Stir and add baked beans and mixed herbs. Season with pepper, chilli powder and Worcester sauce. Simmer for at least one hour.

Serve on jacket potatoes, with rice or on its own with garlic bread.

STEVE CRAM

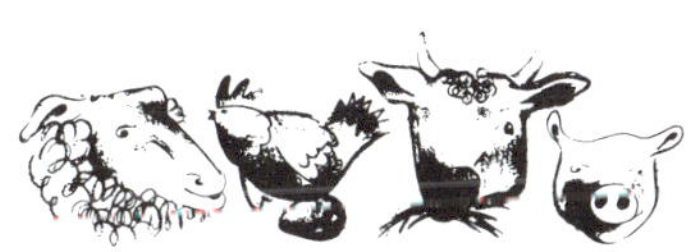

Lamb Chops and Peppers

Ingredients

4 tablespoons oil
4 large loin lamb chops, trimmed
2 onions, thinly sliced
1 garlic clove, finely chopped
1lb tomatoes, skinned and chopped
2 green peppers, seeded and sliced
1 red pepper, seeded and sliced
1 teaspoon crushed coriander seeds (optional)
Salt and pepper
5fl oz dry white wine
1 tablespoon tomato puree

Method

Heat the oil in a large frying pan over high heat, and brown the chops on both sides. Lower the heat, add the onions and garlic. Cover and cook for about 10 minutes or until the onions and garlic are soft and beginning to colour.

Add the tomatoes, peppers, coriander, and salt and pepper to taste. Cover and cook for 15 minutes or until chops are tender.

Remove the chops from the pan and keep warm. Raise the heat and add the wine to the pan. Cook, stirring constantly, until the liquid is reduced by half. Stir in the tomato puree and simmer for 5 minutes. Spoon the sauce over the chops.

Serve with rice, noodles or boiled potatoes.

MIKE NEVILLE, MBE

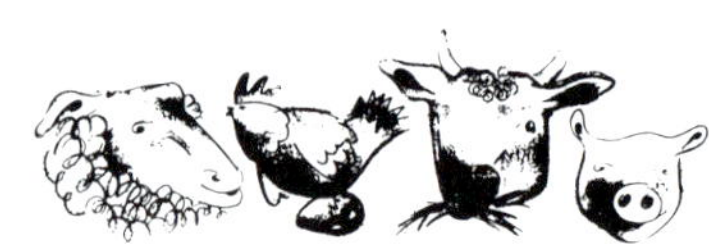

Taffy's Special

Ingredients

1lb mince
2 small onions
1 tin sliced carrots
1 tin garden peas
1 tin sweetcorn
Salt and pepper
1 tablespoon soy sauce
Mixed herbs
Piece of fresh ginger
1 tablespoon sunflower oil
1 tablespoon gravy granules

Method

Dice onions finely and fry until brown and tender. Add the mince, soy sauce, salt, pepper and mixed herbs. Fry until brown. Transfer to saucepan, and add all the vegetables and juice. Bring to the boil then simmer for 10 minutes.

Place the ginger in a piece of muslin and drop into the mixture. Boil for another 20 minutes. To thicken, add about 1 tablespoon of gravy granules and cook for a further 20 minutes.

Take the ginger out and serve on a bed of rice or pasta.

YEOVIL BRANCH

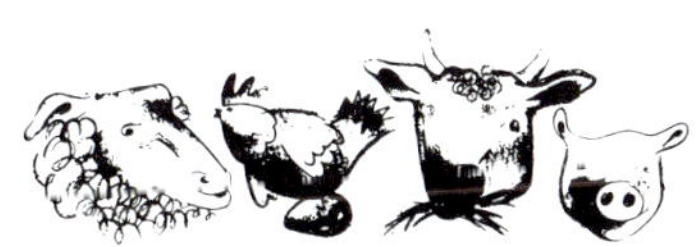

Turkey in Cream and Wine Sauce

Ingredients

1lb turkey breast (or chicken)
2 onions
8oz button mushrooms
1 teaspoon lemon juice
2 tablespoon oil
8oz butter
¼ pint sour cream
2 teaspoon cornflour
1 teaspoon paprika
¼ pint white wine
Salt and pepper

Method

Brown meat in oil. Remove. Melt butter in same pot. Fry onions and mushrooms. Stand for 10 minutes and add the meat. Mix sour cream, cornflour, lemon and paprika. Add to meat and mushroom/onion mix. Add wine. Simmer for a few moments.

Salt and pepper to taste.

Comments

This is a heavenly dish with rice or pasta and green salad.

RAY COONEY

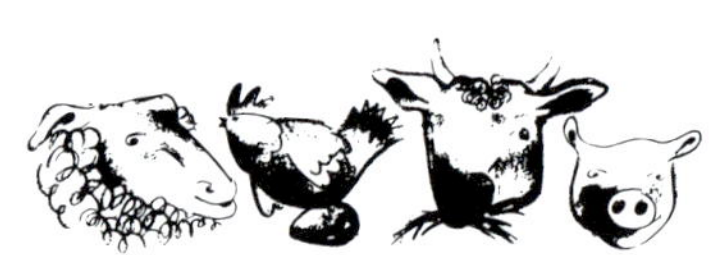

Steak, Kidney and Mushroom Pie

Ingredients

8oz puff pastry
1lb braising beef or chuck steak
3oz kidney
6oz mushrooms
6oz onions
1 tablespoon flour
Pinch dried or fresh mixed herbs
Little stock or water
Salt and freshly ground black pepper
Little dripping or oil for frying

Method

Cube the steak, chop the kidney and onions. In large frying pan, heat dripping or oil and seal the steak and kidney. When brown add the chopped onions. Fry gently for a few minutes then turn into a casserole dish, adding herbs, seasoning and chopped mushrooms. Stir in flour, add stock or water and cook gently in the oven for at least 2 hours at 180°C/350°F (gas mark 4) until tender.

Turn into pie dish, roll out puff pastry about ¼″ thick, cut a strip to fit around edge of pie dish, moisten the edge, press strip on and then put the lid in place, making a hole for steam to escape. Glaze with a little beaten egg or milk, and flute edges with the back of a knife. Bake 30-40 minutes in a hot oven at 220°C/425°F (gas mark 7) until golden brown.

Comments

I give my wife's recipe for steak, kidney and mushroom pie. She is a superb cook and this is one of my favourites.

JIM BOWEN
Central Television

Lamb Crumble

Ingredients

12oz cold roast lamb
3oz onions
4½oz flour
1 level tablespoon tomato puree
½ pint stock
Salt and pepper
2oz butter or margarine
2oz cheese, grated
½ level teaspoon dried mixed herbs

Method

Preheat oven to 190°C / 375°F (gas mark 5). Mince together meat and onions, mix in about ½oz of the flour, the tomato puree, stock, salt and pepper. Turn into a pie dish.

Rub the fat into the remaining flour until it looks like fine bread crumbs. Then stir in the grated cheese, herbs and salt and pepper if required. Spoon crumble mix over the meat. Bake for 45 minutes to 1 hour.

Serves 4.

Comments

This is a good way of using up cold roast lamb. It's cheap and quick to do as well. Nice with baked tomatoes and mushrooms.

LINDA ROY
Carer, Hastings and Rother Branch

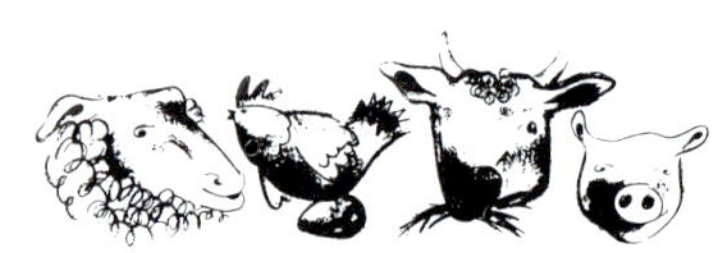

Frosty's Kebabs

Ingredients

8oz boned lamb from shoulder or leg, or beef steak
4 tablespoons plain yoghurt
1½ tablespoons lemon juice
1 cube fresh ginger, peeled and finely grated
1 clove garlic, peeled and mashed to a pulp
1 teaspoon ground cumin seeds
½ teaspoon ground coriander seeds
¾ teaspoon cayenne pepper
¾ teaspoon salt
Vegetable oil

Method

Cut the meat into ¾″ cubes and place in a non-metallic bowl. Put the yoghurt, lemon juice, ginger, garlic, cumin, coriander, cayenne and salt in a bowl and mix well. Hold a sieve over the meat and pour the yoghurt mixture into it. Push mixture through the sieve extracting all the paste you can. Mix the meat and the marinade well, cover and refrigerate for 6-24 hours.

Thread the meat onto skewers and balance them on the rim of a baking tray so that the meat juices drip inside the tray. Brush the kebabs generously with oil and place the baking tray under the grill. When one side of the meat is brown, turn the meat over, brushing with more oil.

PAUL FROST
Presenter, Tyne Tees TV

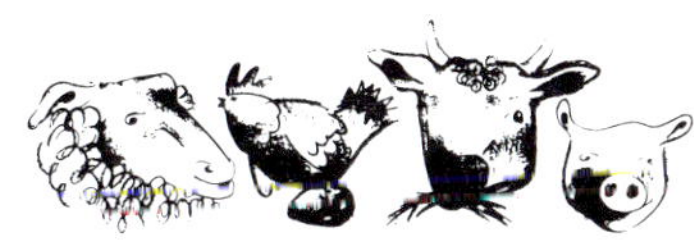

Curried Cider Chops

Ingredients

4 pork chops
¾ pint dry cider
1 egg, size 2
3oz fresh white breadcrumbs
1 level teaspoon chopped sage
1oz butter
1 medium onion, finely chopped
1 level tablespoon curry powder
2 level tablespooons sweet chutney
Salt and pepper

Method

Heat cider in saucepan and reduce volume by one-third. Beat egg and pour it on to a plate, then mix breadcrumbs with sage and salt and pepper on another plate. Trim chops to remove excess fat. Dip each chop first in the egg and then in the breadcrumbs and arrange them in a buttered oven-proof dish.

Melt butter in a frying pan. Fry onion and curry powder until onion is soft. Then stir in chutney and cider and pour the sauce over the chops. Bake in the centre of a moderately hot oven (190°C/350°F/gas mark 5) for about an hour until tender. Serve with duchesse potatoes and salad.

Serves 4.

W. BARTLETT
Buckinghamshire Branch

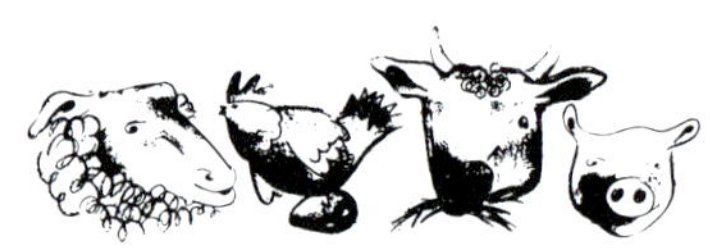

Lamb Kidneys
(COOKED IN BUTTER AND MUSTARD SAUCE)

Ingredients

6 lamb kidneys (can be more or less, depending on your appetite)
Knob of butter
1 tablespoon finely chopped spring onions or ordinary onions
$^1/_3$ cup dry white wine
1 tablespoon Dijon mustard
1 tablespoon butter
Salt
Pepper
Chopped parsley

Method

Melt knob of butter in shallow casserole or deep frying pan. Add kidneys (after removing the outer skin and white fat). Cook on both sides for about 10 minutes, by which time the kidneys should be cooked on the outside and pink in the centre. Remove kidneys to a warm plate.

Add onions to butter in pan and cook for 1 minute. Add the white wine and boil while scraping up the bits on the bottom of the pan. Remove from heat. Add mustard and butter along with salt and pepper to taste.

Slice kidneys about ¼″ thick at a slight angle and add to casserole. Heat over a low heat for a couple of minutes to heat the kidneys through. Add sprinkle of parsley and serve with boiled rice.

Serves 2.

THE RT. HON. DR. DAVID OWEN, MP

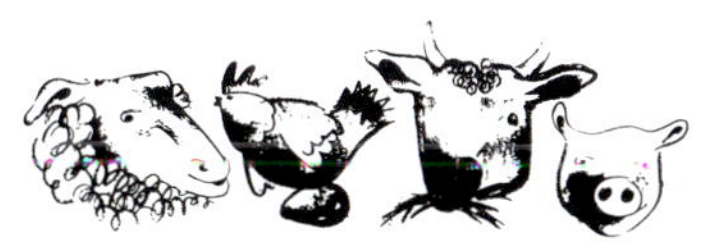

Sweet and Sour Pork

Ingredients

For sauce:

1 tin (13½oz) pineapple
2 tablespoons cornstarch (cornflour)
8oz vinegar
4½oz brown sugar
2 tablespoons soy sauce
2 tablespoons lemon juice
1 small green pepper, coarsely chopped
1 tablespoon pimento, chopped

For pork:

1-1½lbs meat cut into ½″ cubes
3 teaspoons soy sauce
3 tablespoons flour
Fat for deep frying

Method

For sauce:
Drain pineapple chunks, reserve pineapple. Measure syrup. Add water to make up to 8oz liquid. Blend together pineapple syrup and cornflour until smooth. Stir in vinegar, sugar, soy sauce and lemon juice. Cook until thickened and clear. Add pineapple, green pepper and pimento. Mix well. Cover. Simmer over low heat 10-15 minutes.

For pork:
Preheat deep fat until 375°F. Toss pork with 3 teaspoons soy sauce and then 3 tablespoons flour. Fry until cube comes to surface and floats. Add to sauce. Serve with cooked rice.

DR. BRIAN MAWHINNEY, MP
Minister of State for Northern Ireland

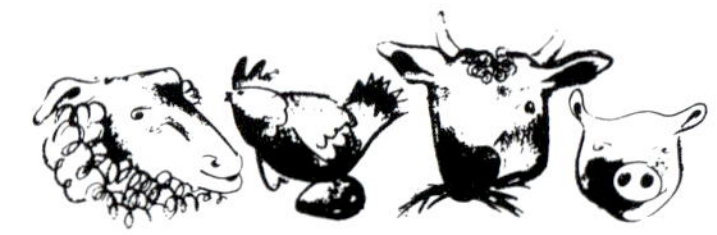

Sid Little's Favourite Curry

Ingredients

2lbs lamb or chicken
1 medium onion per pound of meat
3 cloves of garlic
Small piece of stick cinnamon
Small piece of fresh ginger
½ teaspoon turmeric
½ teaspoon garam masala
1 clove
Fresh coriander
14oz tin of tomatoes, chopped or whole
Salt to taste

Method

Brown the meat or chicken in a little oil, add the chopped onion and fry till golden brown. Grate the ginger and chop the garlic cloves into small pieces, add to the other items, together with cinnamon, turmeric, garam masala, tomatoes, salt, coriander and clove. (Remove clove before serving.) Simmer gently until it is cooked, adding little more water if necessary.

Serve with poppadoms, cooked in ½″ hot oil, and rice, cooked with saffron and turmeric. A nice relish can be made by chopping up half an onion and adding to some tomato ketchup.

SID LITTLE
of 'Little and Large'

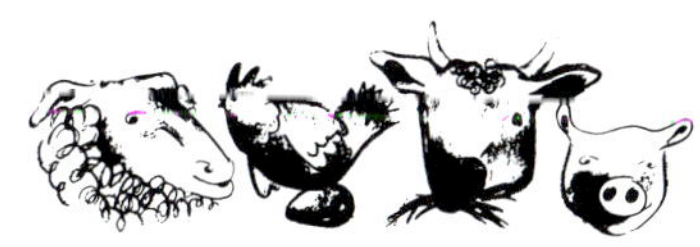

Pork & Apricot Casserole

Ingredients

1lb diced pork
2 tablespoons seasoned flour
2 tablespoons Worcester sauce
2 tablespoons vinegar
2 oz butter
1 can apricot halves
2 tablespoons demerara sugar (if apricots are not in syrup)
2 tablespoons lemon juice

Method

Toss pork in flour. Fry in butter till lightly brown. Drain apricots, reserving juice and chop all but 3. Mix juice with Worcester sauce, sugar, if required, and lemon juice. Add remaining flour to pork and pour in apricot sauce and chopped fruit. Bring to boil. Reduce heat, cover and simmer 45 minutes. Garnish with apricots. Serve with 8oz long grain rice cooked as per packet directions.

Serves 4.

HAZEL TEMPLETON
Harrow & Northwood Support Group

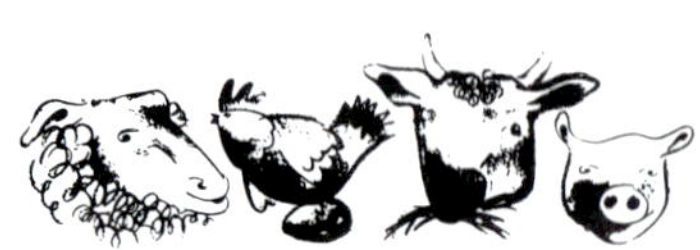

Leek & Bacon Pie

Ingredients

For pastry:
8oz self-raising flour
2oz margarine
Pinch of salt
Cold water

For filling:
1lb leeks
4oz streaky bacon
1 egg
Seasoning to taste

Method

Wash and chop leeks and boil in salted water until just tender. Drain well. Use half the pastry to line a deep pie dish. Chop bacon and mix with leeks, beaten egg and seasoning. Put the mixture in pie dish, cover with remaining pastry, glaze with milk and bake at 220°C/450°F or gas mark 8 for approx 30 minutes until golden brown.

NEATH & PORT TALBOT BRANCH

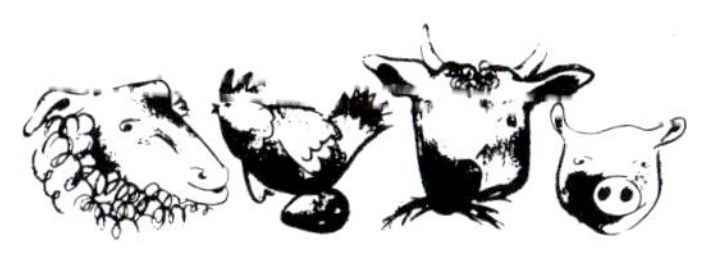

Pasta & Pork Cheese

Ingredients

2oz butter
1 large onion, peeled and thinly sliced
12oz lean minced pork
14oz can tomatoes
1 tablespoon dry sherry
1 clove garlic, peeled and crushed
½ teaspoon dried thyme
1 bay leaf
Salt
Black pepper
1lb frozen whole leaf spinach
6oz noodles
2 teaspoons cornflour

For cheese sauce:
1½oz butter
1½oz flour
¾ pint milk
6oz cheddar cheese, grated

Method

Heat butter and fry the onion till soft. Gradually add the pork and cook until brown. Stir in the tomatoes, add the sherry, garlic, thyme, bay leaf and seasoning. Allow to simmer covered for 30 minutes. Heat frozen spinach with ½oz butter. When soft drain well and spread over the base of a greased oven dish. Cook noodles in plenty of water for 5 minutes. Drain. Add the remaining butter. Blend the cornflour with a little cold water, stir in the pork mixture and bring to the boil.

Then make the cheese sauce: melt the butter, add the flour and cook for a few minutes before adding milk. Bring to the boil. Stir in the cheese and season well. Spoon half the cheese sauce over the spinach. Then top with noodles and the meat sauce. Pour over remaining cheese sauce, sprinkle with grated cheese and bake for 30 minutes at 190°C/375°F (gas mark 5). Serve with salad.

YEOVIL BRANCH

Cobbler's Hot-Pot

Ingredients

1lb loin of pork
1lb carrots
1lb potatoes
1lb pears
Salt
Sugar

Method

Cut the meat into small cubes and peel and core the pears. Cook together in a ½ pint of water for 10 minutes. Transfer to a covered oven dish. Peel and slice the carrots and potatoes and add them to the dish with salt to taste and a little sugar. Cook in a moderate oven for 40 minutes.

Comments

A very simple dish which I found in Germany, where it is called 'Schusterpfane'. Cobbler's Hot-Pot is a close relation of Irish Stew, but the pears give it a unique and lovely flavour. It is an ideal meal for cold weather.

THE RT. HON. LORD WILLIS OF CHISLEHURST

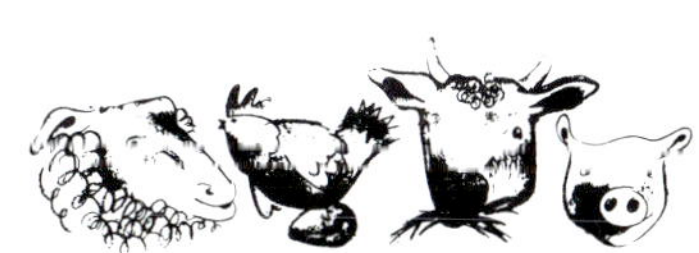

Yorkshire Toad

Ingredients

1½lbs boiled potatoes
2 large sliced onions
1lb pork sausages
Salt and pepper

For batter:
4oz plain flour
1 large egg
½ pint milk
Salt

Method

Slice the potatoes ¼″ thick. Place in baking tin with the sausages and onions, and put into a hot oven. Sieve together the flour and salt into a basin. Add the egg and about half of the milk. Beat well for about 5 minutes. Leave to stand. When the potato mixture has been in the oven for about 20 minutes, add the rest of the milk to the batter, stir well and pour over the top. Return to the oven for 30 minutes until well risen, crisp and brown.

J. BOWKER
York Branch

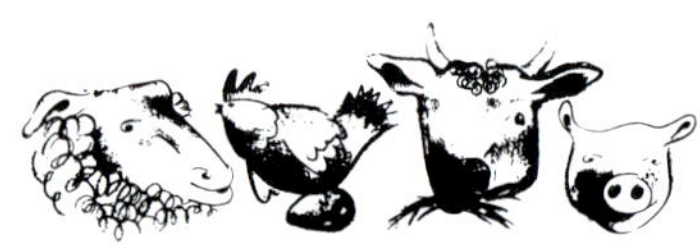

Winter Stew

Ingredients

2lbs good stewing beef, cubed
8oz sliced mushrooms
2 tablespoons oil
1 tablespoon butter
1 tablespoon wholemeal flour
3-4fl oz red wine
¾ pint beef stock
3 tablespoons Worcester sauce
2 tablespoons redcurrant jelly
1 crushed clove garlic
Small pinch of mixed herbs
Salt and pepper

Method

Brown meat in oil and butter. Gradually add flour. Stir well for 1 minute. Add stock slowly, then the rest of the ingredients and simmer for 5 minutes before putting in oven for 3½ hours at 150°C/300°F (gas mark 2).

Comments

I can confirm that it is very good on a cold day.

THE RIGHT REVEREND WILLIAM WESTWOOD
Lord Bishop of Peterborough

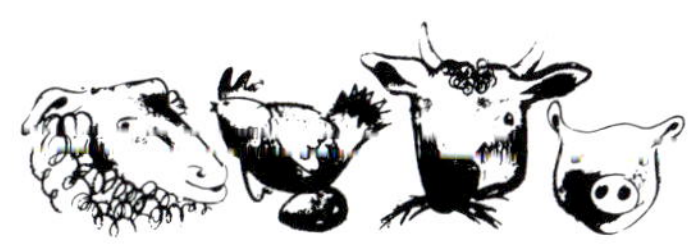

Chinese Pineapple Chicken

Ingredients

4lb chicken (jointed)
4 tablespoons oil
2 garlic cloves
12oz can pineapple cubes
2 tablespoons soy sauce
1 tablespoon sherry
2 pieces stem ginger in juice (drained and sliced)
1 tablespoon cornflour, blended with 2 tablespoons water
Salt and pepper

Method

Heat oil, add garlic and fry chicken pieces till brown. Remove chicken, drain off oil and discard garlic.

Drain pineapple juice into a jug and make up to ½ pint with water. Cut pineapple cubes in half. Put pineapple juice, cubes, soy sauce, sherry and ginger in pan and simmer with chicken joints for 30 minutes. Stir blended cornflour in to thicken, bring to boil, season and serve.

Best served with noodles or rice with fresh mixed green salad.

ELIZABETH, LADY ELLIOT
Oxford

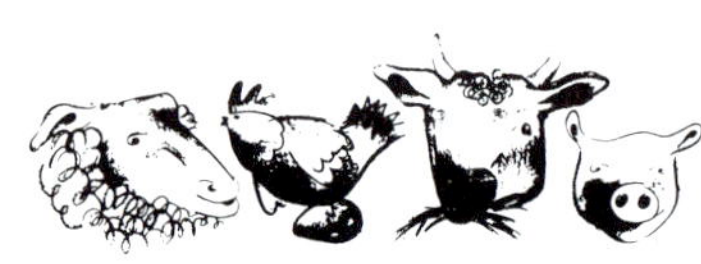

Chicken Indienne

Ingredients

8 good-sized chicken breasts, boned
4 small bananas, finely sliced
24 white grapes, halved and pitted
4 tablespoons crushed hazelnuts
2oz butter
12fl oz basic curry sauce
8fl oz double cream

Method

Remove the fillet (the underside flap) from the chicken breasts. Pound (not too vigorously) each breast and its fillet until flat. Stuff each breast with ½ banana, 6 grape halves and one-eighth of the hazelnuts.

Place fillet on top and fold the ends over and make a rectangular parcel. Place the breasts, rounded side up, close together in a shallow roasting tin in which the butter has been melted. Bake in a preheated oven at 190°C/375°F (gas mark 5) for 20-25 minutes, basting frequently, until cooked through and golden brown.

Make up the curry sauce or use prepared sauce and whisk in the cream. Transfer chicken to a shallow flame-proof dish and pour the sauce over. Cook over gentle heat until bubbling and slightly thickened. Remove from heat and serve.

Serves 8.

ANGELA RIPPON

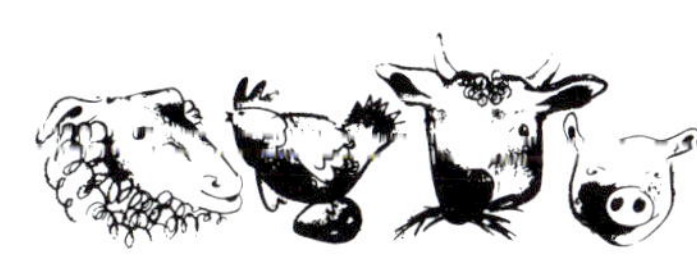

Chicken Cordon Bleu

Ingredients

4 skinless boneless breasts of chicken (about 7oz each)
4 slices cooked ham
4 slices Gruyere cheese
2oz butter
3 tablespoons cooking oil
½ pint beef (yes, beef) stock made with cube
¼ pint Madeira
Black pepper
12 cocktail sticks

Method

Hammer the breasts, not too thin. Cover each one with ham. Cover half of each breast with cheese. Fold over and pin securely with 3 cocktail sticks. Melt the oil and butter in a large frying pan. Fry the breasts quickly on each side, then lower heat and cook for 6 minutes each side and a minute or so up on the folded end until golden brown. Add the Madeira and stock. Simmer for 5 minutes. Take the meat out and keep it hot on your serving dish. Boil the sauce rapidly to reduce the juice. Season. After 4-5 minutes the juice will be quite thick. Take the cocktail sticks out of the chicken, pour the sauce over it and serve.

BONNIE TYLER

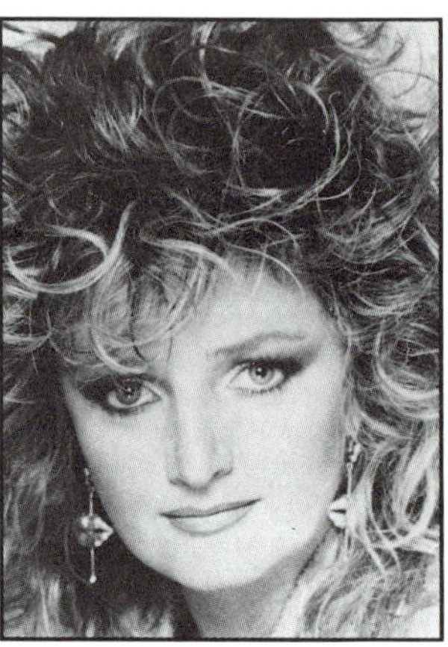

American Chicken Salad

Ingredients

8 chicken breasts
4oz shelled walnuts, inner skin removed
4oz hazelnuts, inner skin removed
Medium Spanish onion
8oz seedless green grapes
4 green eating apples
Celery
Juice of 2 lemons
Fresh tarragon
Lettuce hearts (little gem)
2 bunches watercress
Hellman's mayonnaise (1-2 tablespoons)
Freshly ground black pepper
Sea salt

Method

Gently grill the chicken, retain juices, then pull apart pieces into lengthwise strips rather than cut them. Chop the onion very finely. Chop cored apples lengthwise and sprinkle with lemon juice to stop discolouration. Do not peel. Halve the grapes. Do not peel. Chop best parts of celery into inch-long pieces. Roughly chop the nuts into quarters.

Cover the edge of a large serving dish with lettuce leaves and sprigs of watercress. Mix the chicken pieces into the mayonnaise, add other ingredients, less tarragon, and pile into the centre of the dish. Sprinkle chopped tarragon on top. Serve with new or baked potatoes and with a tomato salad on the side for colour.

MARGARET FRANCE

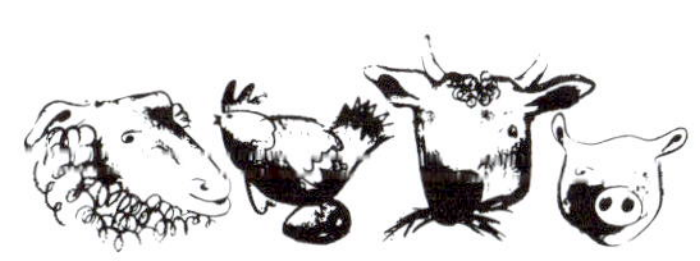

Soloman's Chicken Hot-Pot

Ingredients

- 4 lambs' kidneys, cleaned and sliced
- 1 chicken, jointed, or 4 chicken joints
- 3 medium onions, roughly 10-11oz, chopped
- 5 tablespoons cooking oil
- 3½oz tomato puree (one small tin)
- 2 bay leaves, crushed or cut into small pieces
- 2 teaspoons coriander seeds
- ½ teaspoon each of chilli powder, mixed spice, powdered cinnamon, freshly ground black pepper and freshly grated nutmeg
- 1 tablespoon fresh chopped thyme
- 4 large potatoes, peeled and sliced

Method

Brown the kidneys, chicken and onion in the oil. Place all ingredients except the potato in a casserole, and mix well. Arrange the sliced potatoes neatly over the top. Barely cover with water and cook in the oven at 200°C/400°F (gas mark 6) for 60 minutes. Cover only if it seems necessary.

Serves 4.

RHONA AITKEN
Author of "The Memsahib's Cookbook"

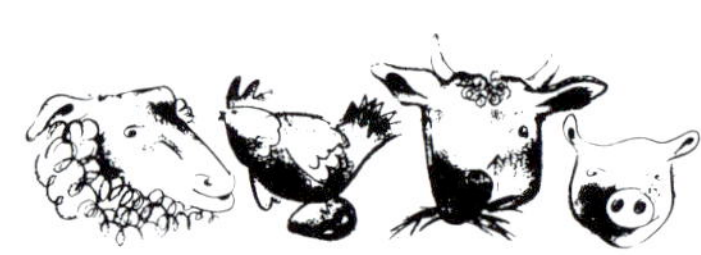

Honeyed Chicken

Ingredients

4 chicken breasts
2 tablespoons honey
1 teaspoon mustard
½ teaspoon tarragon
1 tablespoon tomato puree
¼ pint chicken stock (chicken oxo cube)
Salt and pepper to taste

Method

Place chicken breasts in dish and cook slowly for about 45-60 minutes at 180°C/350°F (gas mark 4) in a small amount of water. Mix together honey, mustard, tarragon, tomato puree, chicken stock and salt and pepper. Pour over chicken. Cook until mixture thickens slightly. Coat chicken with sauce during cooking.

Serve with rice or salad.

CHIEF FIRE OFFICER T. F. ELTON
Tyne and Wear Fire Brigade

Submitted by
HIS WIFE

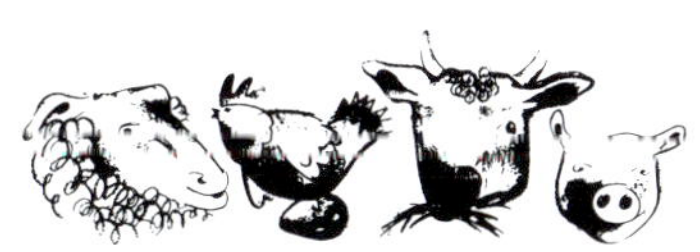

Mexican Chicken

Ingredients

8 chicken thighs
3 tablespoons flour
1 teaspoon salt
1 teaspoon paprika
¼ teaspooon ground black pepper
2oz butter
2 tablespoon oil
1 onion, chopped
3 tablespoons lemon juice
2 tablespoons Worcester sauce
2 tablespoons Tabasco
½ pint water
¼ pint tomato ketchup
1 teaspoon sugar
1 teaspoon chilli powder
¼ teaspoon Oregano

Method

Shake chicken in flour, salt, paprika and black pepper. Brown chicken in foaming butter and oil. Place in baking dish. Add onion to oil and butter and cook until soft. Add all remaining ingredients and cook for 10 minutes over gentle heat. Pour mixture over chicken; cover and bake until tender, keeping well basted.

Serve with rice and green salad.

Comments

This is one of my husband's favourite dishes.

NORMA MAJOR

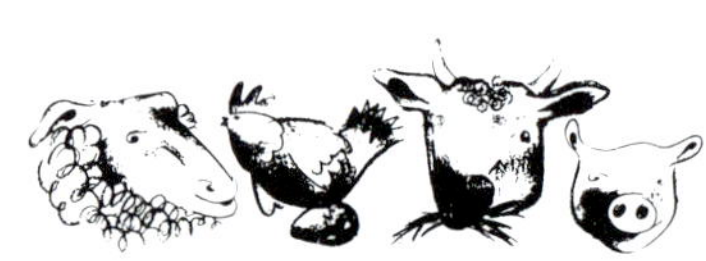

Chicken Dijon
(WITH WINE AND MUSHROOMS)

Ingredients

2 chicken breasts
Olive oil
½ cup white wine
Salt and pepper
1 piece of fresh tarragon or a sprinkle of dried herbs
¼lb button mushrooms

For sauce:
2 teaspoons plain flour
¼ chicken stock cube
½ cup water
1 cup of milk
2 tablespoon cream if available
1½ teaspoon Dijon mustard

Method

Place chicken breasts in a shallow, oven-proof dish and pour a little oil on top and around them. Add mushrooms, wine, seasoning and herbs and cover with tinfoil. When the chicken is cooked – it will take about 45 minutes to cook (200°C / 400°F or gas mark 4) – take it out of the dish together with the mushrooms and place on the tinfoil.

Return the dish with juices to the stove and begin to make the sauce over a very low heat. Mix flour with the stock cube and a little milk to a thin paste in a separate container. Add this to the juices together with the remaining liquids and the Dijon mustard. The cream should be added last. When the sauce looks to be about the right consistency, return the chicken and the mushrooms to the dish and allow them to cook gently for a few seconds before serving.

Serves 2.

PENNY TREADWELL

Rolled Stuffed Chicken

Ingredients

Boned breasts of chicken

Stuffing, as desired

Method

In the middle of chicken breasts there is a little bit of extra flesh. You slice through this, then beat the whole breast out. Mix, or buy, some stuffing to your taste. Spread it over the chicken breasts and roll up longways. Wrap in buttered tinfoil.

Cook in a moderate oven (190°C/375°F/gas mark 5) for 30 minutes.

When they come out they look like a Swiss roll: cut them as you would the same. Serve either hot or cold – if hot with chicken gravy.

BERYL REID

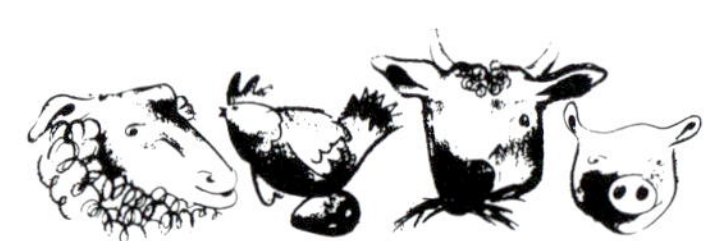

Balinese Chicken and Tomato
(ATAM BUMBU BALI)

Ingredients

2lbs chicken pieces
Salt and pepper
Oil for frying
2 medium onions, finely chopped
2 fresh red chilles, finely chopped
2 cloves garlic crushed
¾ cup tomato puree
2 teaspoons brown sugar
½ teaspoon fresh ginger, shredded
1 teaspoon dried shrimp paste (Blanchen – obtainable from Chinese food stores)
3 teaspoons dark soy sauce
2 cups chicken stock
4 medium tomatoes, skinned and chopped (tinned are fine)
¼ cup thick coconut milk (made by dissolving creamed coconut in hot water)

Method

Season chicken. Fry in hot oil until brown with crisp skin. Drain well and keep warm. Fry onions in 1 tablespoon oil for 3 minutes. Add onions, chilles, garlic and tomato puree and cook on a moderate heat for 5 minutes. Mix brown sugar, ginger, shrimp paste, soy sauce and chicken stock and add to onion mixture. Simmer for 10 minutes. Add chicken and continue simmering until tender. Add tomatoes and coconut milk and cook a few minutes longer.

Garnish with fresh coriander. Serve with rice.

JOHN KEADY

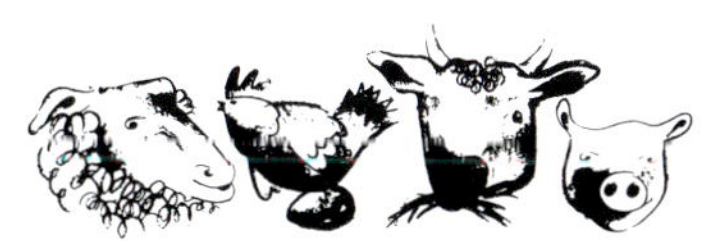

Chicken, Bacon & Mushroom Dish

Ingredients

8 chicken pieces, skinned
8 streaky rashers, de-rinded
4oz mushrooms
4oz butter
1 glass white wine
Small carton double cream
Flour
Pepper
Salt

Method

Lay slices of mushroom on chicken pieces and sprinkle with black pepper. Wrap bacon slice round each one. Put in baking tin with remaining sliced mushrooms over all pieces and dot with butter. Cover with foil and cook in oven until chicken is done. Arrange chicken in oven-proof shallow dish, keep warm. Strain liquid into saucepan, sieve in enough flour and let it bubble to make a wettish paste. Beat in wine and cream alternately to make smooth sauce. Season. Pour over chicken and serve.

Comments

Cook should sip a little wine while making sauce!

EDNA DORÉ
Actress

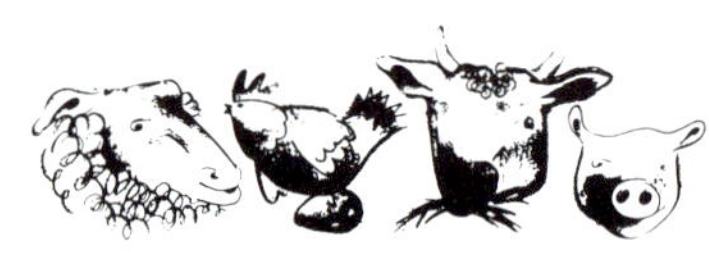

Roast Duck with Marmalade Sauce

Ingredients

1 large duck, 4-5lbs
1 orange
Salt and pepper
6oz fine-cut marmalade
5fl oz orange juice
½ teaspoon sugar
5fl oz chicken stock

Method

Prick duck all over with sharp fork. Halve the orange and place both halves in cavity of the duck. Season skin. Roast, breast side down, on a wire rack over a roasting pan for 40 minutes at 190°C/375°F/gas mark 5.

Turn the duck right way up and smear 1 tablespoon marmalade over the skin. Return to the oven for a final 40-50 minutes. Check near the end of cooking time, and cover with foil if marmalade threatens to burn. Duck should be a rich dark brown. Turn off the heat and let it sit in the warm oven, door ajar, for 5 minutes before carving.

To make the sauce, put the remaining marmalade, orange juice, sugar and stock into a saucepan and bring it gently to the boil, stirring occasionally. Simmer for 10 minutes, making sure sauce doesn't catch on base of pan. Skim and cool. When duck is cooked, reheat sauce and serve immediately.

Serves 4.

MIKE NEVILLE, MBE

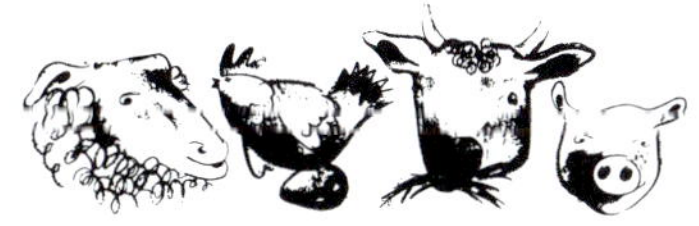

Omelette Cake

Ingredients

4 tomatoes
3 canned artichoke bottoms
2 cooked chicken breasts
5oz butter
3 cloves garlic, crushed
1 large bunch parsley, chopped
Salt and pepper
10 eggs

Method

Peel, de-seed and chop tomatoes, slice the artichokes and chicken meat. Heat 1oz of the butter in a frying pan and fry the tomatoes until brown. Add a little garlic and parsley. Season and leave to cook for about 20 minutes over a low heat. Mix the rest of the parsley and garlic in a bowl and set to one side. Heat 1oz of the butter in a frying pan and brown the artichoke slices. Season and reserve. Brown the chicken in 1oz of the butter and season.

Make 5 small 2-egg omelettes, cooking them one by one in the remaining butter and keep them hot. Place 1 omelette on an oven-proof dish and cover it with chicken. Place the second omelette on top and cover it with fried artichoke. Place the third omelette on top and cover it with garlic and parsley. Place fourth omelette on top and cover it with tomato mixture. Then place the last omelette on top of this. Put the omelette cake in a moderate oven at 160°C / 325°F (gas mark 3) until heated through and serve hot with a curly endive salad.

Serves 6.

SIMON WESTON

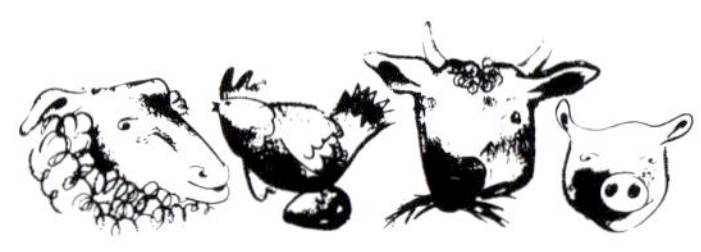

Roast Beef

Ingredients

Joint of rib or topside of beef
Flour
Mustard
Salt and pepper
Olive oil
Cabbage

Method

Prepare the night before: put the flour, mustard, salt and pepper in a frying pan and heat gently stirring all the time. When quite hot add olive oil so the mixture now becomes a paste. Cover the joint with the paste and leave overnight.

Put joint into a preheated oven 200°C/400°F (gas mark 6) for 20 minutes to seal, then reduce heat to 150°C/300°F (gas mark 2). Allow 15 minutes for each pound.

Remove from oven 20 minutes before serving and leave in a warm place: juices will percolate through the joint. Turn the oven up high and cook the Yorkshire pudding and crisp the spuds.

The flour, mustard, etc. left in the roasting dish is now going to make the best gravy you've ever tasted. Add water from cabbage etc. Serve with carrots julienne.

Comments

A proper Yorkshire lunch. Claret through the meal and Camembert with celery will not tax the heart! Bon Appetit!

STEPHEN YARDLEY
Howards Way

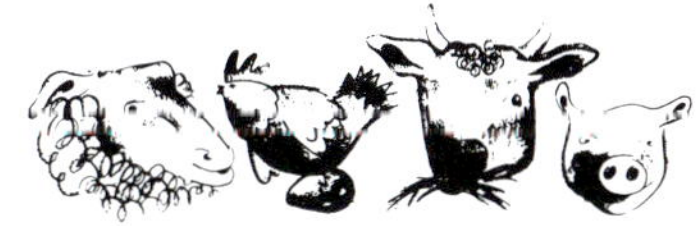

Pseudo Hungarian Goulash

Ingredients

1 large onion
1lb good stewing or braising steak
1 tin Italian plum tomatoes
2 teaspoons paprika

Method

Fry the onion in butter and remove from the pan. Cut up the steak into bite-sized pieces and seal in the pan. Add paprika and the tin of tomatoes. Cover and cook very gently until tender – usually about 1½-2 hours.

This should be served with dumplings but is equally good with boiled potatoes and colourful vegetables.

MARY LUCAS
Seaford

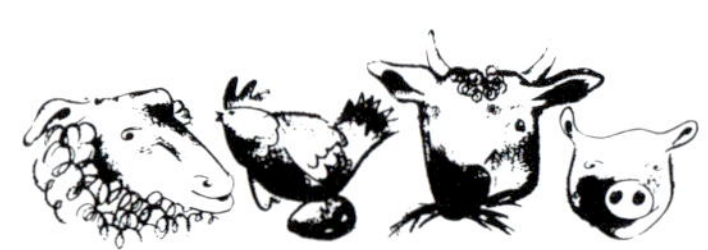

Devonshire Pan Pie

Ingredients

1lb lean minced beef
1 large onion, sliced
3 large carrots, diced
Salt and pepper
1 beef stock cube
Shortcrust pastry

Method

Dissolve beef stock cube in a pint of boiling water and add minced beef, onion, carrots and salt and pepper. Place in a saucepan and cook on a slow heat for 45 minutes.

Make up enough short crust pastry to cover top of saucepan, using the lid as a cutter, and place on top of other ingredients. Cook for 30 minutes with saucepan lid in place; then remove lid and place pan under the grill for a few minutes to brown top of pastry.

TORBAY BRANCH

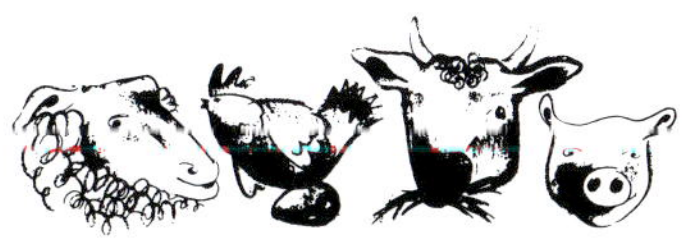

Easy Casserole

Ingredients

1lb beef, cut in cubes or minced
1 medium sized onion, chopped
1 small tin crushed pineapple
1 packet instant tomato soup
Water to mix
Extras such as cooked carrot, peas or celery if you like

Method

Put all ingredients in a casserole. Bake in oven at 150°C/300°F (gas mark 2) for 2 hours. Thicken before serving, if necessary.

GRACE DU FAUR
ADARDS, New Zealand

Meat Casserole Dish

Ingredients

To any casserole dish using pork, beef or lamb, add Ginger Beer with the stock. Gives a delicious flavour.

A GENTLEMAN CARER
Bideford, Devon

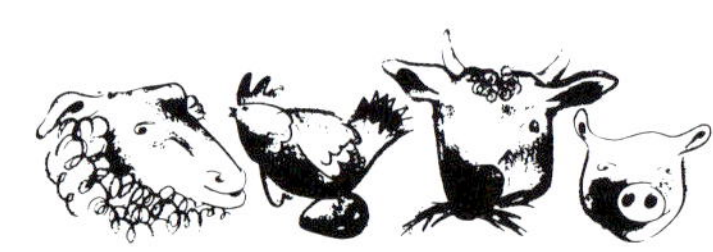

Parcel Cooking

Ingredients

2 small lamb chops
1 medium potato
1 small onion
1 small carrot
A little butter or fat of your choice
Salt and pepper

Method

Place all the ingredients on a sheet of baking foil. Add fat and seasoning and wrap up as a parcel. Place on baking tray and then put into a moderate oven for 1 hour.

Comments

This is more an idea than an actual recipe. I consider to be ideal for a person living alone as it is a complete meal, easily prepared with no saucepans to wash afterwards.

CHERRY MARR, CPN

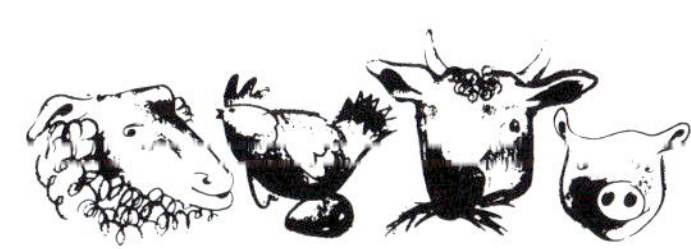

Pork Chop Casserole

Ingredients

Pork chops

For every 2 chops allow:
1 large apple
1 large onion
1 dessertspoon demerara sugar
Sprinkling of sage

Method

Peel and slice the apple, put it in a greased casserole and sprinkle it with sugar. Slice the onion, sprinkle it with sage and put it with the apple. Brown the chops quickly and put in casserole. Season to taste. Cover tightly with greased lid. Cook in moderate oven 180°C/350°F (gas mark 4) for 1½-2 hours.

Serve with jacket potatoes baked in the oven at the same time.

THE RT. HON. LORD MURRAY OF EPPING FOREST AND LADY MURRAY

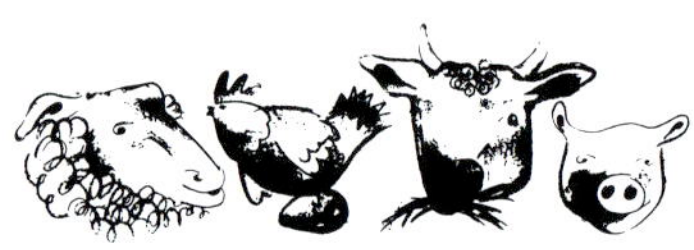

Margaret Foster's Chicken

Ingredients

6 chicken pieces
1 small tin condensed chicken soup
1oz sultanas
Pinch of mixed herbs

Method

Place chicken pieces in casserole and cover with chicken soup. Add sultanas, herbs and seasoning to taste. Cook in oven at 220°C/425°F (gas mark 7) for 30 minutes, followed by a further 30 minutes at 200°C/400°F (gas mark 6).

Serves 6.

Comments

A very easy dish, but tasty!

JANE McADOO

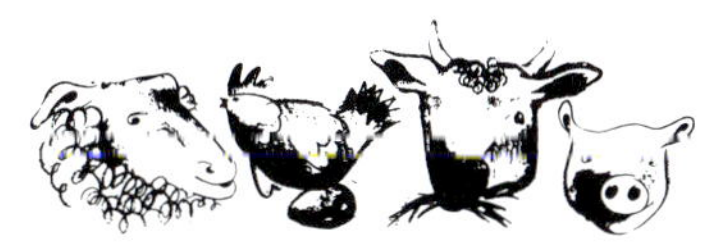

Stuffed Marrow

Ingredients

Marrow
Onions
Tomatoes
Salt and pepper
Sausage meat

Method

Peel marrow, slice in half lengthways, remove pips. Line each half with onion, then a layer of tomatoes, and a layer of sausage meat. Put halves together, fasten with string and roast until brown and crisp. Mince can also be used.

WINNIE EWANS
National Office, Alzheimer's Disease Society, Balham

Pork Swiss Style

Ingredients

2 lbs pork fillets (tenderloin)
3oz plain flour
6oz butter
2 finely chopped onions
½ pint white wine
8oz mushrooms
½ pint cream
1 tablespoon chopped parsley

Method

Cut meat into strips. Dip in seasoned flour. Fry meat and onions in 4 oz butter. Add wine and cook to smooth consistency. Set aside. Fry mushrooms in rest of butter. Stir in cream and parsley. Add meat and onion mixture, stir well.

B. M. PURDUE

Devilled Chicken

Ingredients

4 pieces chicken

For sauce:

2 tablespoons Mango chutney (or Branston)
1 tablespoon malt vinegar
2 tablespoons oil
1 tablespoon Worcester sauce
2 teaspoons English-made mustard
¼ teaspoon paprika
Pepper to taste
½ teaspoon salt
½ teaspoon mixed herbs

Method

Mix together sauce ingredients, pour over chicken and cook in oven until tender.

ELIZABETH WEAVER

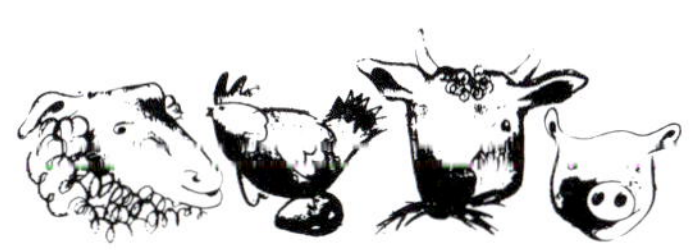

Sussex Chicken

Ingredients

2 chicken portions
½-1 packet plain crisps
2oz strong cheese, grated
2oz low fat margarine
Salt and pepper

Method

Skin and season chicken portions. Crush crisps and mix with cheese. Melt margarine and dip chicken portions in this, then in the cheese and crisp mixture, coating well. Arrange portions in an oven-proof dish and pour remaining melted margarine over chicken. Bake uncovered in the middle of the oven at 190°C/375°F (gas mark 5) for 40-45 minutes.

AUDREY MUNRO

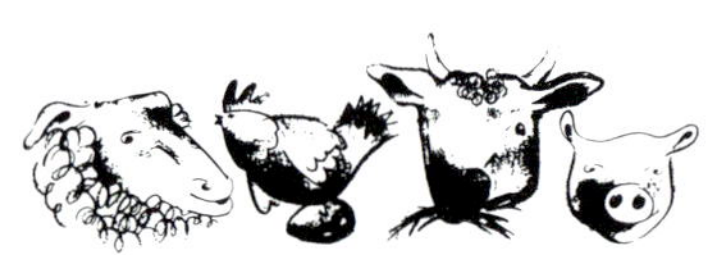

Supper Dishes

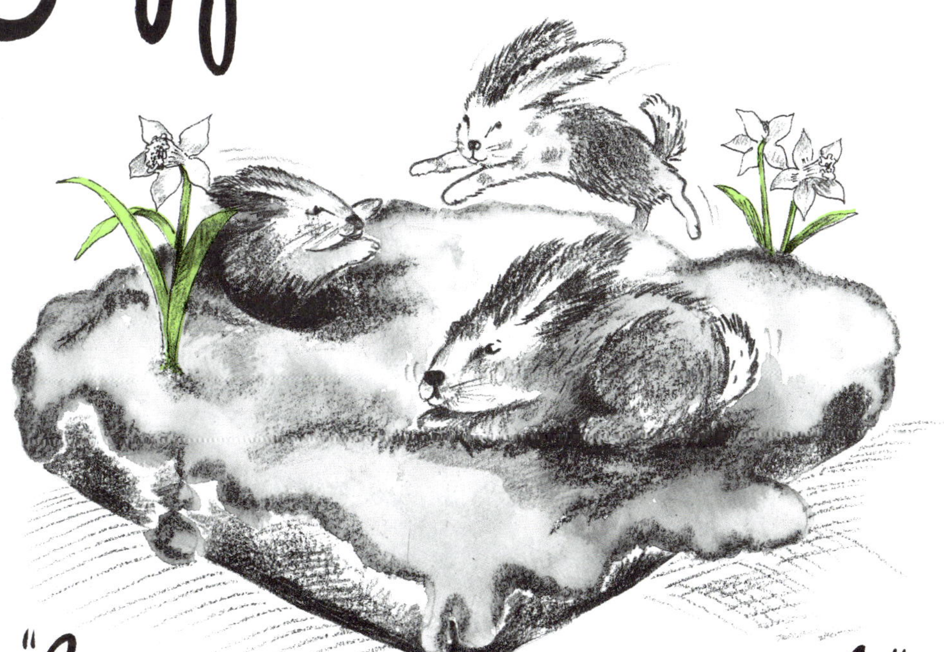

"A warren of Welsh Rarebits"

Eggplant Parmesan

Ingredients

3 large aubergines, peeled and cut into ½″ slices
1 egg
8fl oz milk
Fine white breadcrumbs or cornmeal
1-1½lb mozzarella, sliced
3-6oz Parmesan, grated

For tomato sauce:
Olive oil
1-2 large onions, chopped
4-7 cloves garlic, minced
2-2½ pints tinned tomatoes, drained
Big squeeze tomato puree
4fl oz white wine
Handful fresh basil
2 teaspoon fennel seeds
Salt and pepper

Method

Heat oil and fry onion and garlic until soft. Add tomatoes and cook for 10 minutes. Add everything else for the sauce and simmer for an hour, until thick. Sprinkle aubergines with salt and leave for 30 minutes. Rinse and dry. Beat egg and milk together. Pour crumbs on to a large plate. Heat oil as high as it will go without smoking. Dip aubergine slices in eggy milk, then crumbs, then fry a few at a time until browned. Drain well.

Cover bottom of large rectangular dish with some tomato sauce. Follow with a layer of aubergine, more sauce, a layer of mozzarella and a generous sprinkling of Parmesan. Continue layering until you finish with a final generous dusting of Parmesan covered very lightly with some sauce. Bake at 180°C/350°F (gas mark 4) for up to an hour, until bubbling and browned.

MARGARET FORSTER
Author

Cauliflower Foogath

Ingredients

1½lb cauliflower
4 tablespoons cooking oil or ghee
8oz onion, chopped
1½″ fresh root ginger, peeled and very finely chopped
1 teaspoon ground tumeric, or 3-4 teaspoons chopped fresh turmeric (see *Comments*)
6fl oz coconut milk, fresh, tinned or reconstituted from dessicated coconut

Method

Separate the cauliflower into sprigs and chop any excess stalk into small pieces. Heat the oil in a large saucepan and fry the onion until brown. Add the ginger and turmeric, followed by the cauliflower. Mix well and then pour in the coconut milk. Cover and simmer for 6-7 minutes, then remove the lid and give it a good stir. Continue cooking for a further 3-4 minutes – the cauliflower should be still a little crisp. Serves 4.

Comments

I have made this dish with potato, and found it very interesting. Fresh ginger has a lovely flavour which is quite different from dried, and it seems to complement vegetable dishes. If you search, you might be able to get hold of fresh turmeric – known as Indian saffron – and a rhizome rather like ginger. It has a lovely flavour, and is especially nice served chopped and raw in salads.

RHONA AITKEN
Author of "The Memsahib's Cookbook"

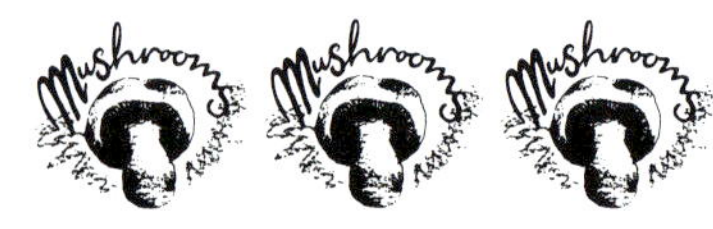

Baked Egg & Bacon

Ingredients

1-2 tablespoons olive oil
4 tablespoons chopped bacon
4 tablespoons chopped parsley
4 eggs
4 tablespoons double cream
Salt and pepper

Method

Heat the oil in a frying pan and sauté the bacon until crispy. Drain it well on kitchen paper and mix with the chopped parsley. Add seasoning to taste.

Sprinkle the base of each ramekin dish with a little of the bacon mixture and break an egg carefully into each one. Bake in the oven for 12-15 minutes or until the whites are just setting and the yolks are runny.

Swirl cream over the top of each egg and serve immediately.

THE RT. HON. SIR PETER MORRISON, MP

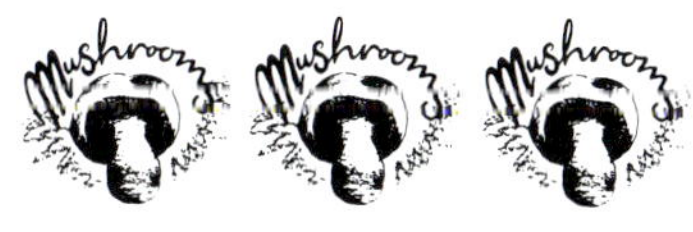

Italian Rice Salad

Ingredients

8oz brown rice
2 free-range eggs
7oz tuna fish
2oz gruyere cheese
Yellow or red pepper
Small bunch fresh basil or parsley
2 tablespoons cold-pressed mayonnaise

Method

Wash rice and place in saucepan with 2½ times its volume of boiling water. Cook for 25-30 minutes. Drain and allow to cool. Hard boil the eggs, cool and shell. Slice or chop the eggs. Drain the oil or brine from the tuna fish and flake. Dice the cheese into small squares, and wash and finely dice the pepper. Finely chop the basil or parsley, reserving a few sprigs for decoration. Mix all the ingredients together with the mayonnaise. Place in serving dish and decorate with basil, parsley or pepper.

Comments

This was always one of the house standbys during my childhood. I love this recipe simply because it is easy to make, and then keeps magnificently in the fridge for quite a few days. It makes an excellent starter to any meal, or makes a whole meal in the summer. All you have to do is add different kinds of mayonnaise to alter the taste. One can also be imaginative and switch cheeses or use tinned sardines instead of tuna, for example.

Tips: An olive oil and cider or wine vinegar can be used in place of mayonnaise. Use one third vinegar to oil and season to taste with freshly ground black pepper, sea salt and a pinch of dry mustard powder. Shake well before dressing salad.

KATIE BOYLE

Diet Pasta

Ingredients

8oz cooked pasta (approx 4oz uncooked weight)
6oz tomatoes, chopped
3oz onion, peeled and chopped
2oz courgettes, sliced
1 teaspoon tomato puree
1 teaspoon dried thyme, oregano or basil
5oz chopped cooked ham or skinned chicken
2oz Edam cheese, grated
Pepper

Method

Place vegetables, herbs, tomato puree and pepper in a saucepan. Add cold water to come halfway up vegetables. Bring to boil, stir and simmer for approx 5 minutes. Add meat and stir to heat through. Add pasta and stir again. Add more water if the mixture seems dry. Bring to boil and remove from heat. Pour into round or oval oven-proof dish and top with cheese. Place under hot grill and cook until cheese is melted and brown. Calories per portion: approx 355. Serve with braised celery or grilled tomatoes.

Serves 2.

Comments

Different combinations of vegetables can be used depending on availability and choice. Likewise the herbs and pasta can be varied.

J. E. WILLIAMS
Mid Sussex Branch

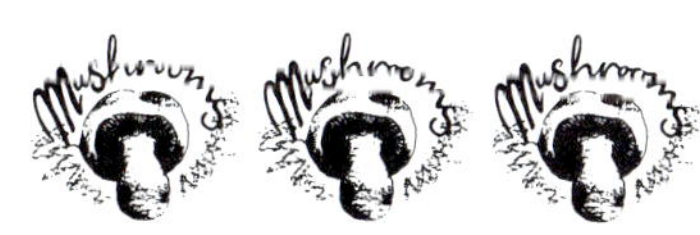

Cold Egg Dish

Ingredients

4 hard boiled eggs
½ pint double cream
¼ pint Maggi aspic jelly (1 dessert spoon aspic powder)
2 teaspoons Worcester sauce
2 teaspoons essence of anchovies
1 flat teaspoon curry powder
¾ flat teaspoon salt (or little more)
Pepper to taste

Method

Take the yolks of 3 boiled eggs and mash with the Worcester sauce, essence of anchovies, curry powder, salt and pepper. Beat up aspic jelly (made day before with gill of water). Add this to the egg mixture. Beat the cream, not too stiff, and fold in.

Put in fridge for 2-3 hours. Serve in a souffle dish decorated with one hard boiled egg cut into slices.

Comments

A bowl of lettuce with French dressing is good with this dish.

JANE GOW, DBE
Widow of Ian Gow, MP

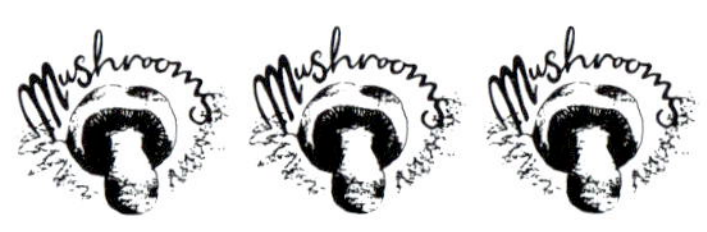

Savoury Supper Dish

Ingredients

1 medium-sized potato
1 medium-sized onion
1oz plain flour
1 egg
3 rashers bacon
Salt and pepper

Method

Cut the bacon into small pieces and fry lightly. Grate the potato and onion into a bowl and add the egg and flour and stir well. Add the bacon and seasoning. Heat some fat in a frying pan until just hot, then spoon in the mixture and cook for 6-8 minutes, until golden brown. Turn the mixture over and fry the other side for 6-8 minutes. Serve with mixed vegetables or a salad.

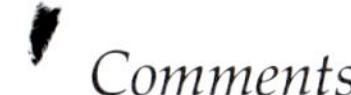

Comments

Vegetarians may substitute sweetcorn for the bacon.

MARY CALLAND
Rhyl and District Branch

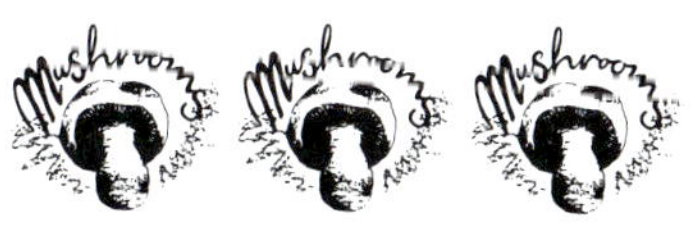

Bacon Pancake

Ingredients

3oz plain flour
½ pint milk
2 eggs
Salt and black pepper
1½ level teaspoons mixed herbs
8oz streaky bacon
1oz dripping

Method

Sift flour into a bowl and stir in half the milk. Add the eggs and remaining milk and whisk until the batter is smooth and light. Season with salt and ground pepper and mix in the herbs.

Remove the rind from bacon and cut rashers in half inch wide strips. Fry over medium heat for 3-4 minutes. Measure 2 tablespoons of the fat into a heated fireproof dish, add drained bacon and pour over the pancake batter. Bake in the centre of a pre-heated oven at 180°C/350°F (gas mark 4) for 30 minutes or until set. Serve with grilled tomatoes.

THE RT. HON. BARRY JONES, MP
Shadow Minister of State for Wales

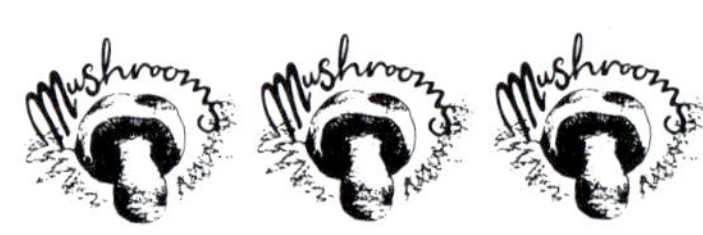

Sausage & Leek Supper

Ingredients

1½lb potatoes, peeled and sliced
1oz butter
1lb sausage (with herbs, optional), sliced
1 onion, sliced
4 leeks, cleaned and sliced
1½oz flour
¾ pint fresh milk
4oz cheese, grated
1oz fresh breadcrumbs

Method

Cook potatoes in boiling salted water for 5-10 minutes. Melt butter in a large pan, add the sausages and cook for 5 minutes. Add the onion and leeks, cook for a further 5 minutes. Add the flour, cook for 1 minute. Gradually add the milk and 3oz cheese. Bring to the boil and simmer for 1-2 minutes, stirring. Transfer to an oven-proof dish, arrange potato slices on top, sprinkle over the breadcrumbs and remaining cheese and bake at 200°C/400°F (gas mark 6) until browned.

KAY O'SHEA
Merseyside Branch

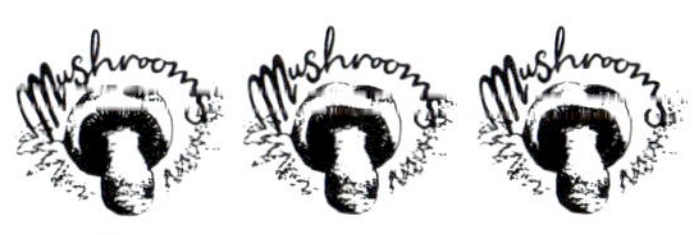

Ham & Banana in Cheese Sauce

Ingredients

4 slices ham
4 peeled bananas
1 heaped tablespoon plain flour
1 heaped tablespoon butter
½ pint milk, warmed
4oz grated cheese (strong cheddar) or 3oz Parmesan
Breadcrumbs
Extra butter
Extra grated cheese

Method

Grease an oven-proof dish. Wrap each banana in a slice of ham and lay them in the dish. Make a béchamel sauce, add the cheese and pour over. Melt extra butter in a saucepan, add breadcrumbs and extra grated cheese. Spread over top of bananas. When required bake in oven at 180°C/350°F (gas mark 4) until browned for about 30 minutes.

Comments

This can be made with leeks or chicory instead of bananas (poach them until tender first) or with leeks and/or chicory, omitting the ham if you are a veggie person.

PRUNELLA SCALES
Actress

Scrambled Eggs & Smoked Salmon on Toast

Ingredients

8 pieces of thick sliced brown bread
6 jumbo eggs
1 dessert spoon cottage cheese
1 small knob butter
3 slices smoked salmon

Method

Break eggs and whisk in a bowl with butter and cottage cheese. Place in microwave for 2-3 minutes (depending on microwave wattage). Toast bread; butter, cut into triangles and place all around the edge of an oval plate. When eggs are ready place in the middle of the plate and place thinly cut strips of salmon across and diagonally on top of the eggs. If you don't have a microwave then cook the eggs in a pan on the hob as you would with normal scrambled eggs.

Comments

This is supposed to feed four but if you're starving you could eat the lot yourself.

PAULINE DANIELS
"Slap and Tickle Enterprises"

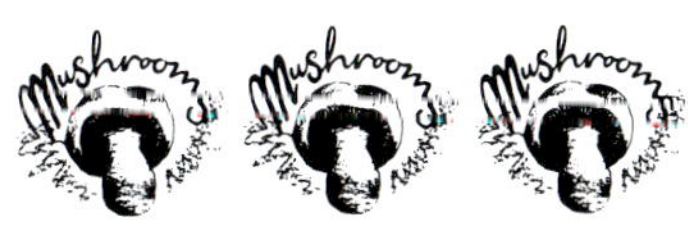

Cheshire Fitchet Pie

Ingredients

2lb potatoes, mashed
8oz onions
1lb baking apples
1lb streaky bacon*
2-4oz Cheshire cheese
2-3oz butter
Milk

* Vegetarians can substitute baked beans for bacon.

Method

Grease an oven-proof dish. Fill with alternate layers of previously cooked bacon, apples, onions and ending with mashed potatoes. Sprinkle generously with Cheshire cheese. Bake for 20 minutes in a moderately hot oven. It is important to keep everything moist so use plenty of butter to cook onion and use plenty of milk and butter when creaming potatoes.

Serves 4-6.

Comments

This old Cheshire dish was served to farm labourers as a harvest feast.

GLADYS ASTBERY

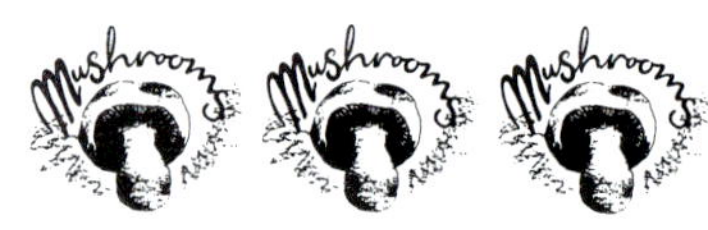

Easy Pizza

Ingredients

For filling:
12oz tin of tomatoes
1 large onion
1 clove garlic
1 tablespoon soy sauce
1 tablespoon tomato puree
1 teaspoon Italian seasoning or other mixed herbs
Salt and pepper
Oil for frying
6oz cheese

For base:
8oz flour
1 teaspoon baking powder
¼ pint milk
4 tablespoons vegetable oil
Anchovies and black olives for decoration

Method

Slice the onion and fry with the crushed garlic over a gentle heat until soft. Cut up the tomatoes and add them with their juice. Fry gently mashing the tomatoes as the mixture cooks. Add herbs, soy sauce, tomato puree and seasoning. Continue to cook until the mixture thickens. Turn out onto a plate and leave to cool.

Sift flour and baking powder and salt. Add milk and oil. Knead until smooth then spread onto an oiled baking sheet or two 8″ tins. Put some grated cheese on top, and spread the tomato mixture over this. Add more cheese, and decorate with anchovies and olives if wished. Bake in a hot oven 230°C/450°F (gas mark 8) for about 25 minutes or until dough is cooked, and the cheese is bubbly. You could add bacon, ham, mushrooms, peppers etc. to the topping.

JOAN M PLATTS
Watford

Favourite Tomato Snack

Method

On a round of hot buttered toast, spread Marmite sparingly, cover with thinly sliced cherry tomatoes, and top with Hellman's mayonnaise. Do not attempt to eat this with your fingers, otherwise it will collapse.

Comments

In these days of quality control, tomatoes seem to have lost their taste almost entirely. If, however, you grill them, somehow the original tangy taste of childhood reasserts itself. A quick alternative to cooking is my favourite tomato snack.

IAN McKELLEN

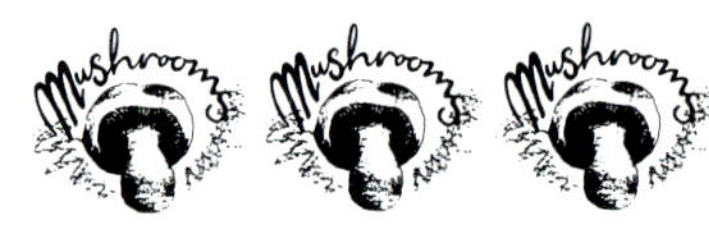

Vegetarian Slimmers' Spaghetti

Ingredients

1 or 2 packets Philadelphia light cream cheese
1 packet frozen creamed spinach
1 packet spaghetti

Method

Defrost the spinach by warming gently in pan. Add cheese and mix. Add salt and pepper to taste.

Comments

Delicious served with spaghetti. Equally good on toast. Would be good to fill vol-au-vents.

M. JENKINS
Southwark Branch

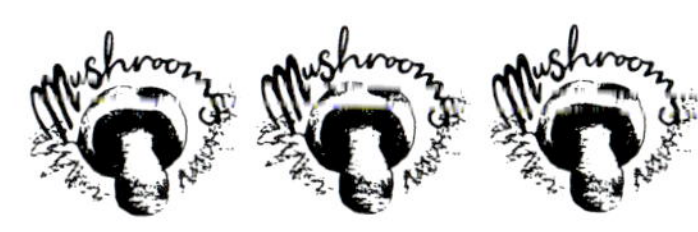

Polly's Scramble

Ingredients

1 finely chopped onion
4 rashers diced lean bacon or diced ham
4 large tomatoes, skinned and chopped
3-4 eggs
Salt and pepper
Paprika
1 tablespoon chopped parsley
A little butter or margarine

Method

Cook onion in butter until tender and add tomatoes and meat for a further 2-3 minutes. Stir the beaten eggs into the mixture and season to taste. Continue cooking, stirring occasionally, until the eggs are just set.

Serve on toast sprinkled with parsley and a little paprika.

Comments

This is only the basis. Add anything you like – peas, mushrooms, even cooked, diced potatoes.

POLLY HEMMINGWAY and ROY MARSDEN

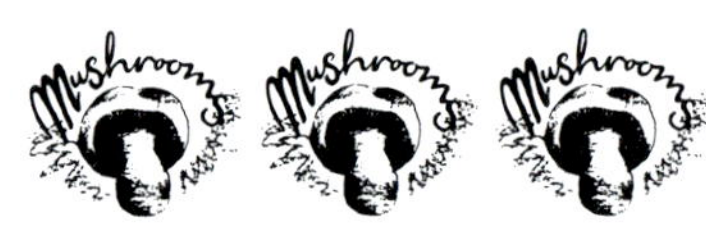

Spinach Roll

Ingredients

½ packet puff pastry
1lb frozen spinach
6oz Cheshire cheese
2 eggs
Little salt and black pepper

Method

Thaw pastry if frozen. Cook spinach in as little water as possible and drain very well. Beat eggs. Grate cheese into large bowl, add spinach, salt and pepper and most of beaten egg.

Roll pastry to large square. Spread filling over one half, fold over other half and seal edges with water. Brush top with egg and make a few cuts with a sharp knife. Bake at 200°C/400°F (gas mark 6) for about 30 minutes.

JUDITH SKINNER

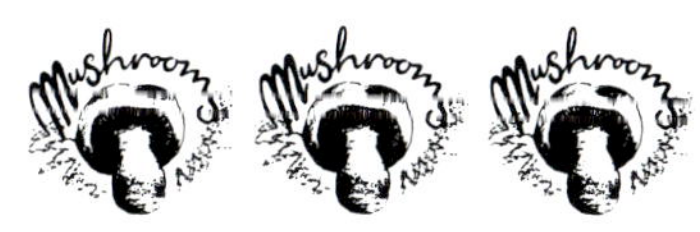

Toasted Philly

Ingredients

Streaky bacon (if possible, maple-cured and unsalted)
Two slices bread
Tomato chutney
Philadelphia cream cheese

Method

Bake bacon in oven, until crisp and brown. Spread one side of each slice of bread with chutney; spread cheese quite thickly on top of chutney. Place bacon on top of cheese.

Sandwich both together and cook in toasted sandwich maker.

Comments

A quick favourtie recipe that I can give to Sir Geoffrey after a late night sitting.

ELSPETH HOWE

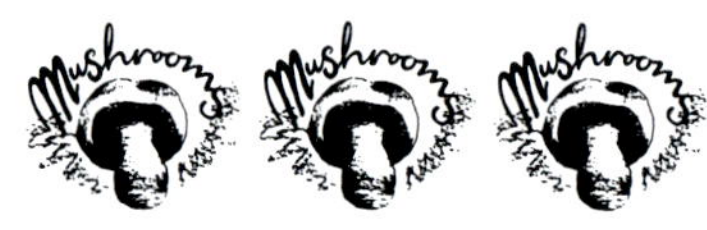

Cottage Cheese Griddle Cakes

Ingredients

1 small carton cottage cheese
1 tablespoon melted butter
2 large eggs
2oz self-raising flour
1 tablespoon milk

Method

Put cottage cheese in bowl. Gradually mix in melted butter and whisked eggs. Stir in flour and milk, mixing to a thick batter. Drop spoonfuls on to a hot well greased frying pan. When one side is browned, turn over and cook the other side. Keep hot, and serve with a few rashers of tasty bacon and sausages.

CHRISTINE WHILD

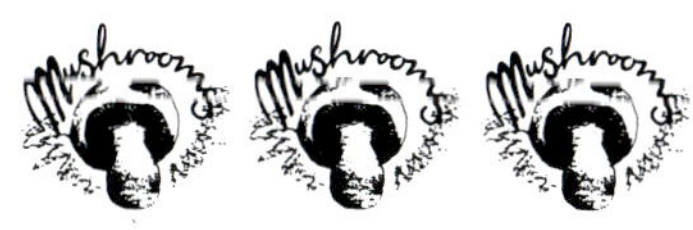

Maltese Eggs

Ingredients

Tomatoes
Onions
Oil
Salt and pepper
Curry powder
Eggs

Method

Take equal quantites (by weight) of tomatoes and onions. Peel and chop them finely. Stew slowly in oil until they make thick puree. Season with salt and pepper and curry powder (approx 1 dessertspoonful for each 1lb vegetable), and cook, stirring, for further quarter of an hour. Beat 1 egg per person and add, stirring well with fork. When mixture is ready, no trace of egg should be visible. Eat very hot.

DAWN MARRIOTT

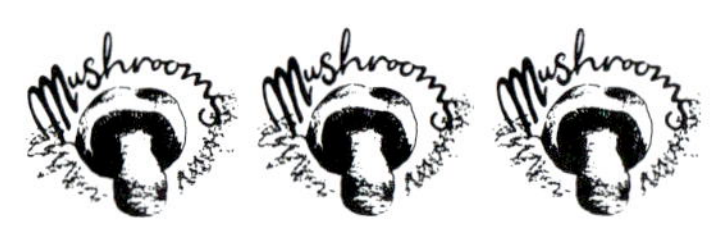

Terribly Easy Ham & Chicory
(IN RICH CHEESE SAUCE)

Ingredients

Chicory
Butter
Lemon juice
Ham
Cheese sauce

Method

Parboil, or better still braise gently in butter and lemon juice, 1 large or 2 small heads of chicory per person. When tender but still firm in the middle, drain and wrap each head in a slice of ham from which the fat has been removed. (The cheapest supermarket pack is perfectly adequate.) Lay the bundles side by side in an oven-proof dish. Pour over your best cheese sauce to cover and sprinkle a bit more grated cheese over the top. Bake in the oven until browned and bubbling – about 45 minutes at 190°C/375°F (gas mark 5).

Comments

Serve with hot crusty bread or, better still, warmed cheese straws.

CLIFF MICHELMORE
Broadcaster

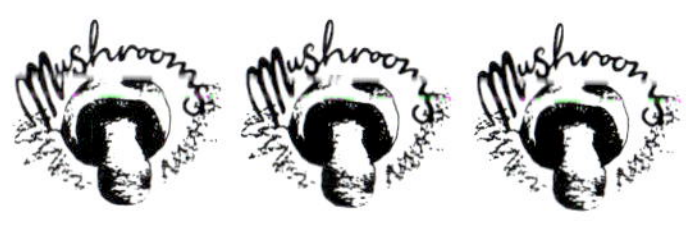

Savoury Potato Cakes

Ingredients

7oz can pork luncheon meat
8oz mashed potato
1 dessertspoon chopped parsley
1 tablespoon tomato ketchup
1 egg
Crisp brown breadcrumbs for coating and a little fat or oil for frying

Method

Chop the luncheon meat finely and mix with the parsley and ketchup and mashed potato.

With floured hands, form into round cakes. Brush with beaten egg and coat with the browned crumbs then fry in the hot fat until crisp and brown on both sides.

Serves 4.

TORBAY BRANCH

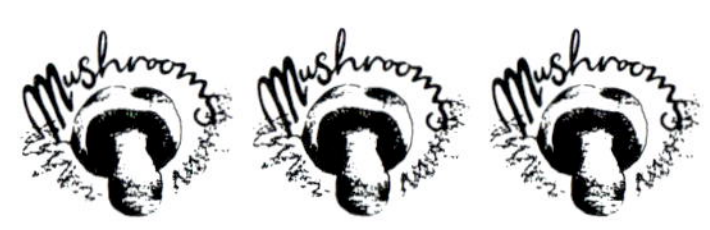

Stuffed Ham Slices

Ingredients

Asparagus, banana or parboiled leek

Cheese sauce

Method

Wrap 3 or 4 asparagus spears (or a banana or leek) in a slice of cooked ham. Cover with cheese sauce. Bake for approximately 30 minutes at 200°C/400°F (gas mark 6).

Multiply the ingredients by the number in your family or the number of guests!

Leek & Potato au Gratin

Ingredients

Potatoes
Leeks

Cheese sauce

Method

Thinly slice approximately equal amounts of potatoes and leek – amounts dependent upon appetite and number of persons. Boil for about 10 minutes. Place into a greased pie dish and cover with a fairly thick cheese sauce. Bake for 20 to 30 minutes at 200°C/400°F (gas mark 6).

Both recipes by:
ENID STOCKWELL

Eggy Bread

Ingredients

1 egg
3 tablespoons milk
2 slices bread
Pinch of salt

Method

Beat together the egg, milk and salt. Pour the egg mixture over the two slices of bread on a flat plate. Allow the bread to soak up the egg for about 5 minutes, turning if necessary.

Fry in a little vegetable oil until brown, turning once. Allow to cool slightly and cut into fingers.

The fingers can then be spread with a little Marmite or golden syrup or eaten as they are.

Comments

Fingers suitable for fingers!

ANN BLOFIELD

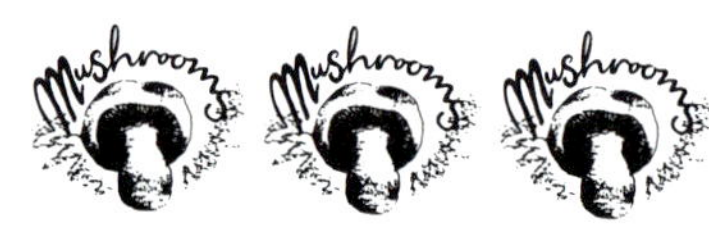

Selsey Rarebit

Method

First take a slice of bread (I prefer white) and toast one side. Butter the untoasted side and add grated or chopped cheese, some cut peppers if available, a little chopped onion if you like (I usually don't), salt and pepper to taste and, if you like, a little tomato, sliced. Then put back under the grill, and grill it until it bubbles. It is now ready.

Comments

Clap two of these together, face to face, and it is transformed into a MARTIAN PANCAKE.

Not very original, I suppose, but I like it!

PATRICK MOORE
Astrologer

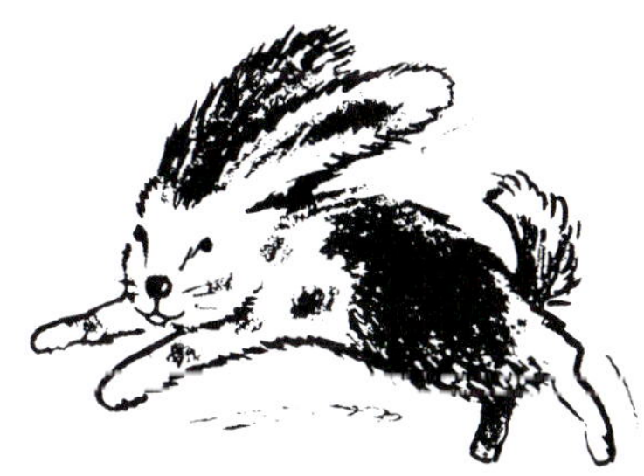

Welsh Rabbit
(RAREBIT)

Ingredients

4 teaspoons butter or margarine
1lb shredded sharp Cheddar cheese
¾ teaspoon Worcester sauce
½ teaspoon salt
½ teaspoon paprika
¼ teaspoon dry mustard
¼ teaspoon cayenne pepper
2 eggs, lightly beaten
1 cup flat beer or ale, at room temperature. *NB U.S. cup – ½ pint*

Method

To be cooked in a microwave oven.

Melt butter in a 2 quart casserole or bowl for about 1 minute. Add cheese, Worcester sauce, salt, paprika, dry mustard and cayenne. Mix thoroughly. Cook, covered, for 3 minutes stirring at 1½ minutes. Stir a little of the hot cheese mixture into beaten eggs and then blend slowly with hot mixture and stir briskly. Gradually stir in beer and mix well. Cook, covered, for 6 to 7 minutes, stirring at 2 minute intervals. Remove from oven and beat briskly with a whisk to blend thoroughly.

Serve over crisp toasted French bread slices and garnish with tomatoes.

ALAN AYCKBOURN

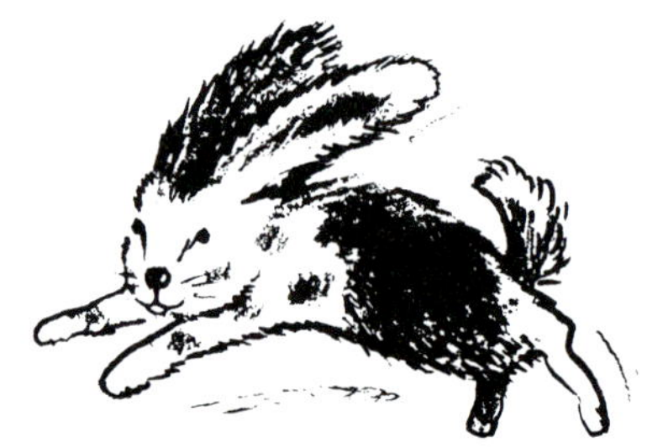

Welsh Rarebit

Ingredients

2 slices wholemal bread – each ½″ thick
Cayenne pepper
Mustard
Grated cheese

Method

Lightly toast one side of each of the slices of bread. Sprinkle the other side of bread with cayenne pepper to taste, or lightly spread with mustard.

Add ¼″ layer of finely grated cheese – any sort will do but use organic cheese if you can get it.

Place under a low grill until the cheese is golden brown on top. Serve and eat while piping hot.

DAVID BELLAMY

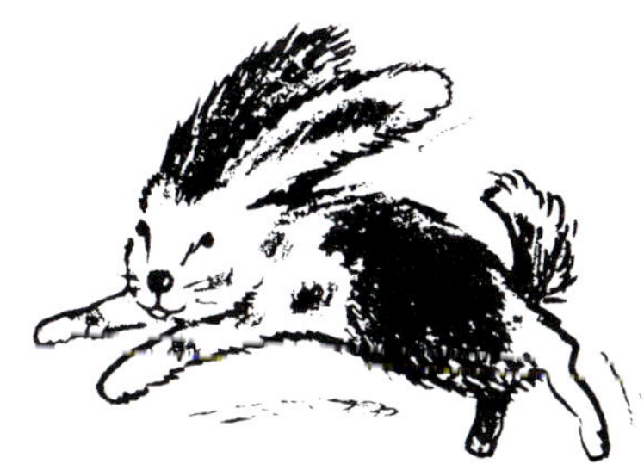

Favourite Recipe for Welsh Rarebit

Ingredients

4oz fresh Cheddar or Cheshire cheese
½ teaspoon dry mustard
A little paprika
Few grains of cayenne pepper
Salt
A little beer or stout
Hot buttered toast

Method

Shred the cheese and put it in a double boiler. Let it melt slowly over hot water kept just under boiling point. Add the mustard, paprika, cayenne and salt to taste according to the needs of the cheese. Then stir in gradually as much beer as the cheese will absorb. The mixture should be smooth and velvety.

Serve on hot buttered toast or hot toasted biscuits.

THE RT. HON. DAVID STEEL, MP

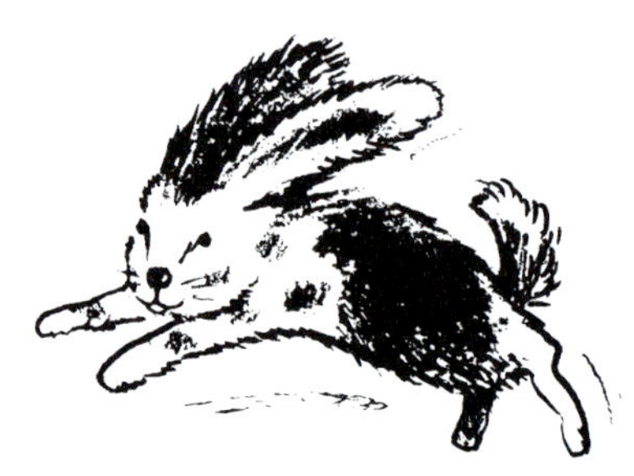

Salads

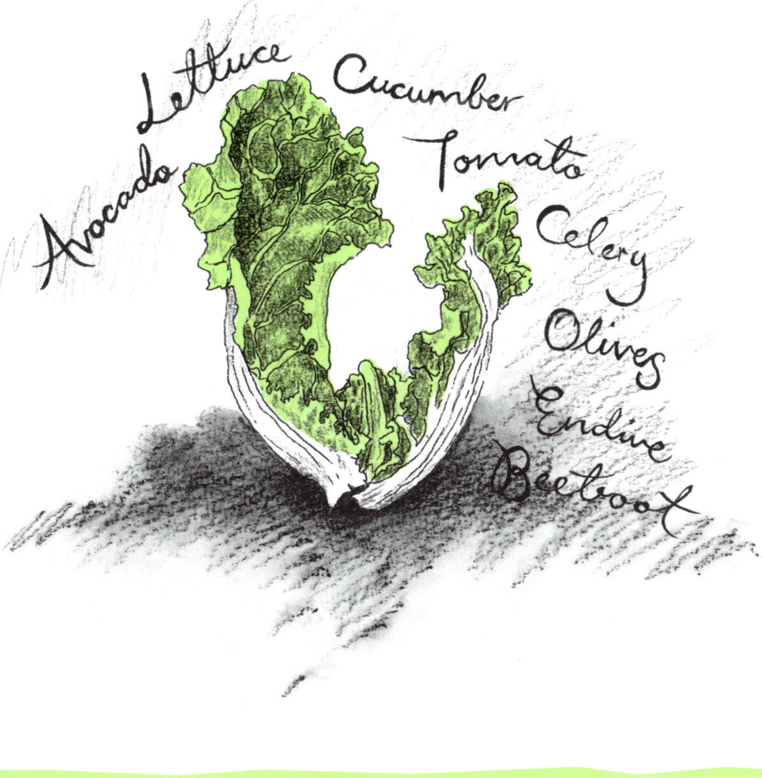

Lettuce
Cucumber
Avocado
Tomato
Celery
Olives
Endive
Beetroot

Rainbow Flower Salad

Ingredients

4 leaves of curly endive, broken into even-sized pieces
1 small head of radicchio, broken into even-sized pieces
2 medium-sized cooked beetroots, cut into bite-sized chunks
4″ piece of white radish, scraped and cut into several chrysanthemums

6 spring onions, trimmed
8 radish roses
4 cherry tomatoes, skinned
1 large carrot, scraped and chopped

Method

Arrange all the ingredients attractively on one or two plates.

To make chrysanthemums, take a walnut-sized piece of radish and make cross cuts as close together as you can, without cutting through to base. Sprinkle with salt, easing it gently between the cuts. Leave for 30 minutes, then rinse and carefully open slits. Radish roses are made by cutting a row of petal shapes around a radish using a sharp knife, keeping them joined at the base. Cut more rows of petal shapes between and above the first row and continue cutting until you reach the top of the radish. Place in iced water for several hours to open out.

ROSE ELLIOT
From 'St Michael Vegetarian Cookery'

Submitted by
JILL SUDBURY
Marlborough Support Group

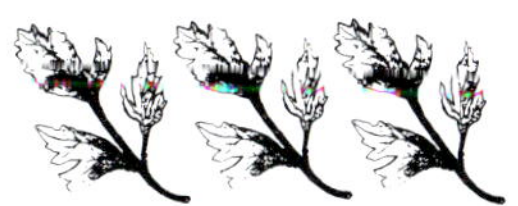

Winter Slaw

Ingredients

1lb brussel sprouts
8oz grated carrots
1 sliced head celery
3oz chopped nuts

For dressing:
½ pint natural yoghurt
¼ pint low-cal mayonnaise
2 teaspoons whole grain mustard
Salt and pepper

Method

Trim sprouts and shred finely in processor. Mix together all salad ingredients and season. Mix dressing ingredients, pour over salad and toss well to coat. Cover and chill thoroughly before serving.

Comments

Fresh beansprouts and/or a diced apple/peas make tasty additions to this salad. Don't worry about the sprouts! Once shredded nobody can ever guess the 'secret' ingredient.

BARBARA HEWITT
Jersey Broadcaster

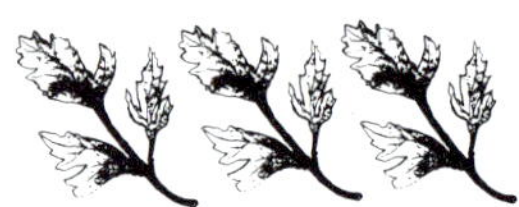

Herby Cream Cheese Salad

Ingredients

7oz cream cheese
5 tablespoons chopped fresh mixed herbs
Crisp lettuce
Plain flour (for dusting)

For dressing:
3 tablespoons olive oil
1 tablespoon white wine vinegar
½ teaspoon English-made mustard
Salt and pepper

Method

Make dressing. Spoon-cut cream cheese into 20 small pieces and roll into balls with floured hands. Spread herbs on plate and roll cheese balls to coat. Refrigerate for 30 minutes. Dip lettuce leaves in dressing to coat. Divide lettuce between 4 plates and place 5 herb-coated balls in the centre of lettuce.

Serves 4.

COLCHESTER STANWAY TOWNSWOMEN'S GUILD

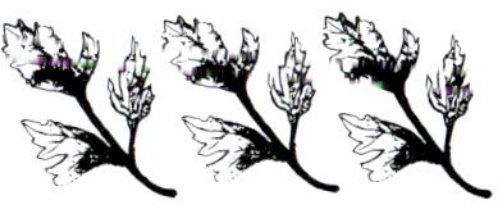

Overnight Layered Salad Cake

Ingredients

1 medium-sized iceberg lettuce
A bunch of spring onions
8oz can water chestnuts
½ red or green pepper, seeded
2 stalks celery
10oz packet frozen peas
½ pint mayonnaise
1 teaspoon sugar
4oz grated Parmesan cheese
1 teaspoon salt
¼ teaspoon garlic powder
¾lb bacon, crisp fried and drained
3 hard-boiled eggs
2 tomatoes

Method

Wash lettuce, drain and slice up coarsely. Spread lettuce over bottom of a wide, deep serving dish. I use a glass fruit bowl. Slice spring onions and sprinkle over lettuce. Drain water chestnuts and slice. Sprinkle over onions. De-seed the pepper and slice in long slices and sprinkle over chestnuts. Slice celery and sprinkle over pepper. Open packet of frozen peas. Sprinkle with sugar, Parmesan cheese, salt and garlic powder and add to salad. Finely chop the bacon and sprinkle over salad. Coarsely chop up boiled eggs and sprinkle over salad. Cover and chill overnight. Just before serving cut tomatoes into wedges, and arrange around the top. Use a spoon and a fork to serve. Portions should include some of each layer.

Serves 8-10 people.

MARIAN DAVIES
Singer/T.V. Presenter/Journalist

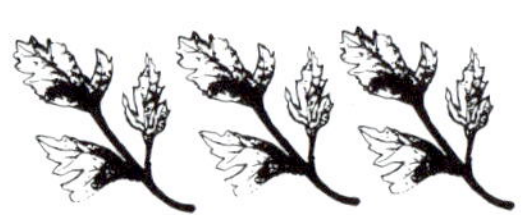

Potato Salad

Ingredients

2lb Jersey new potatoes – mids/Royals
3 tablespoons vinaigrette dressing
8oz streaky bacon
3 hard-boiled eggs
½ bunch sliced spring onions
2 bunches trimmed watercress
2 tablespoons fresh chopped parsley

For dressing:
¼ pint Jersey whipping cream
1 tablespoon lemon juice
1 tablespoon mild mustard (wholegrain is excellent)
1 teaspoon caster sugar
1 tablespoon wine/tarragon vinegar
Salt and freshly ground black pepper

Method

Cook the potatoes (in their skins) in boiling salted water until just tender. Drain and immediately toss in vinaigrette dressing (the potatoes will soak up the dressing easily when very hot). Leave to cool. Grill bacon until very crispy. Crumble. Roughly chop eggs. Mix together potatoes, bacon, egg, spring onions, watercress and parsley.

For dressing:
Put all ingredients in a screw-top jar and shake well to mix. Pour over salad, toss well and chill before serving.

BARBARA HEWITT
Jersey Broadcaster

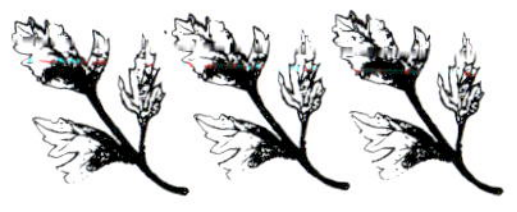

Cottage Cheese Salad

Ingredients

2 large bananas
1 large avocado
1 large green apple

8oz cottage cheese
Iceberg or other lettuce and watercress for base

Method

Slice the bananas into thick chunks. Peel the avocado, remove the stone, cut the fruit into thick wedges. Slice the apple.

Pile the cottage cheese on a base of coarsely shredded lettuce. Arrange watercress sprigs around the edge. Pile the prepared fruit on top. Eat at once.

Comments

The banana, avocado and apple will keep their colour if you squeeze a drop of lemon juice on them first. Any fruit is nice in this kind of salad. Nuts sprinkled on top go well too.

I look upon the kitchen as a tiled cell – everything I make is quick and easy!

CARLA LANE
Television Scriptwriter

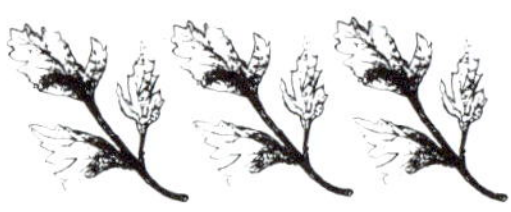

Vegetarian & Vegetable Dishes

Lentil Cheese Loaf

Ingredients

6oz lentils
4oz Cheddar cheese, grated
1 onion, chopped
Salt and pepper, freshly ground to taste
1 teaspoon dried herbs (rosemary or sage or thyme)
2oz fresh breadcrumbs
1 egg, beaten
1½oz butter or margarine

Method

Pre-heat the oven to 180°C/350°F (gas mark 4) and lightly grease a 1lb loaf tin. Wash the lentils twice in cold water and drain them well. Cover them with twice their volume of cold water in a large saucepan, cover and bring to the boil. Reduce the heat and simmer the lentils for 20 minutes, until they are quite soft.

Mix the cheese, onion, salt, pepper and herbs with the cooked lentils. Add the breadcrumbs, egg and butter to the lentil mixture and stir well. Add more breadcrumbs if the mixture is sloppy.

Press the mixture into the loaf tin, and bake for 40-45 minutes. Turn out onto a platter and serve hot.

Serve with a vegetarian gravy or tomato sauce or cheese sauce, and a green salad.

Comments

Good source of protein and calcium.

LINDA McCARTNEY
From her own cookbook

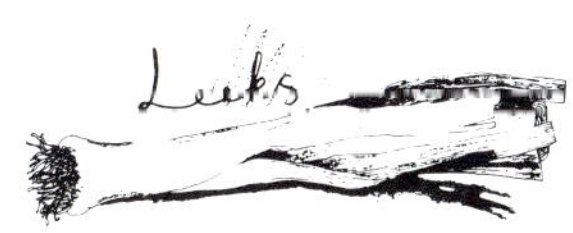

Potato Galette

Ingredients

1½lb potatoes, peeled
5oz cheese, grated
1 egg, beaten
Margarine
1 onion, chopped
Salt and pepper

Method

Boil the potatoes and mash together with margarine and seasonings. Mix in the remaining ingredients except for 1 oz cheese.

Flatten out in an oven-proof dish, sprinkle the remaining cheese on and bake for 30 minutes at 200°C/400°F (gas mark 6).

Garnish with slices of tomato and serve while hot.

BARNSLEY BRANCH

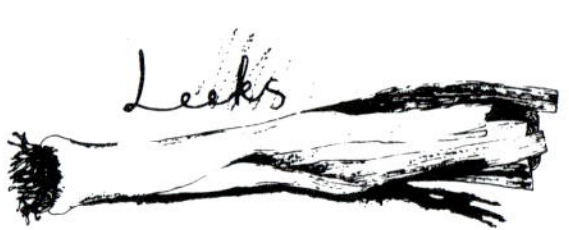

Vegetable Bake

Ingredients

1oz margarine
1oz flour
1 pint milk
Salt and pepper
Pinch of nutmeg
2oz cheese, grated
1lb onions, thinly sliced
2lb potatoes, peeled and thinly sliced*
6oz mushrooms, sliced
1 stick celery, chopped
5fl oz single cream

* I sometimes replace 8oz potatoes with sliced carrots

Method

Melt the margarine in a pan, stir in flour and cook gently for 1 minute, stirring. Gradually stir in milk. Bring to boil and continue to cook, stirring, until sauce thickens, then add seasoning to taste. Combine the vegetables with the sauce and turn into 2 pint oven-proof casserole. Pour over the fresh cream and bake in oven at 180°C/350°F (gas mark 4) for about 1¼ hours. Remove from oven and scatter top with grated cheese. Return dish to oven for about 15 minutes until vegetables are cooked.

Serves 6.

CAROLE LAMB
Yeovil Branch

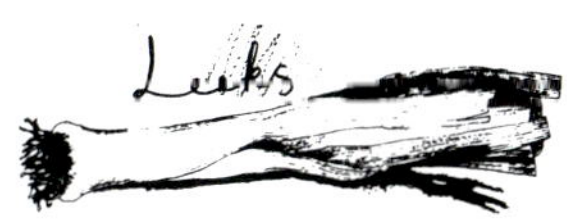

Flaky Mushroom Roll

Ingredients

½oz butter or margarine
1 onion, peeled and chopped
8oz mushrooms, wiped and chopped
2 tablespoons chopped fresh parsley
4oz brown rice, cooked
Salt
Freshly ground black pepper
Little raw egg yolk
Sprigs of parsley to garnish

For rough puff pastry:
8oz fine ground wholemeal flour
1 teaspoon salt
2 teaspoons lemon juice
6oz hard butter or block margarine from the refrigerator
About 8 tablespoons cold water

Method

Preparation time: 40 minutes, plus chilling. Cooking time: 30 minutes – oven: 220°C/425°F (gas mark 7).

First make the pastry. Mix the flour and salt in a large bowl and grate the butter. Add the lemon juice and water, then mix quickly to a fairly soft dough. Gather this in to a ball, wrap in cling film and chill for at least an hour. Roll the dough into an oblong. Mark this lightly into 3 equal sections, then fold the bottom third up and the top third down, to make layers. Seal the edges by pressing them lightly with your rolling pin to trap the air, then give the pastry a quarter turn.

Repeat the rolling, folding and turning four times.

continued

Flaky Mushroom Roll (cont.)

Method (cont.)

Heat the butter or margarine in a large saucepan and fry the onion and mushrooms quickly over a high heat for 2-3 minutes. Remove from the heat, add the parsley, rice, salt and pepper and leave to cool.

Divide the pastry in half, then roll each piece into a rectangle 30 × 25cm (12 × 10 inches). Place one of these rectangles on a baking sheet, carefully spoon the mushroom mixture on top, and brush the edges with cold water. Put the second piece of pastry on top and press edges together, then trim. Make a few holes for the steam to escape, and brush with egg yolk.

Bake in a pre-heated oven for 30 minutes. Serve garnished with sprigs of parsley. Serve also with RAINBOW FLOWER SALAD (see Salads Section).

ROSE ELLIOT
From 'St Michael Vegetarian Cookery'

Submitted by
JILL SUDBURY
Marlborough Support Group

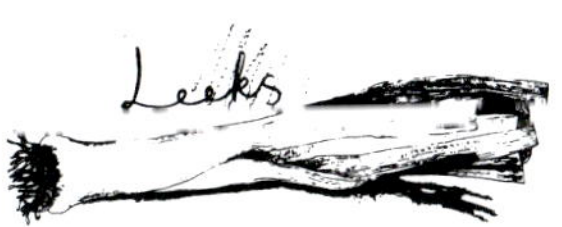

Filled Pancakes

Ingredients

½ pint batter
1oz butter
1 small finely chopped onion
½ crushed clove garlic
8oz mushrooms
Lemon juice
Salt and pepper
¼ pint single cream
1 tablespoon plain flour
Grated cheese

Method

For filling:
Sauté the onion, garlic, mushrooms with the butter and lemon juice. Add the flour and single cream.

Make pancakes and fill with mixture. Place in a dish. Dot with butter and grated cheese and place in a hot oven for 10 minutes.

THE RT. HON. PAUL CHANNON, MP

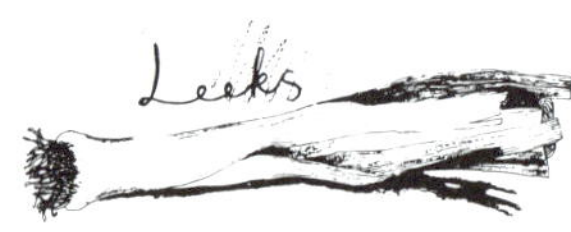

Wyau Sir Fon
(ANGLESEY EGGS)

Ingredients

6 medium-sized leeks
2 tablespoons butter
2oz plus 2 tablespoons grated Cheddar cheese
8 hard-boiled eggs
1lb hot mashed potatoes
Salt and pepper to taste
1 tablespoon flour
½ pint warm milk

Method

Clean the leeks and chop them into pieces, then cook them in boiling salted water for 10 minutes. Strain very well and add them to the hot mashed potatoes. Add half the butter, season to taste and beat or liquidise until it is a pale green fluff. Arrange around the edge of an oval or round oven-proof dish and keep warm.

Heat the other tablespoon butter, stir in the flour and add the warmed milk, stirring well to avoid lumps. Put in the 2oz grated cheese and mix well. Cut up the eggs and arrange in the middle of the leek and potatoes and cover with the cheese sauce. Sprinkle the remaining cheese on top and put into a hot oven 200°C/400°F (gas mark 6) until the top is golden brown.

Serves 4 or less as it's too delicious to share!!!

JOHN MARLOW

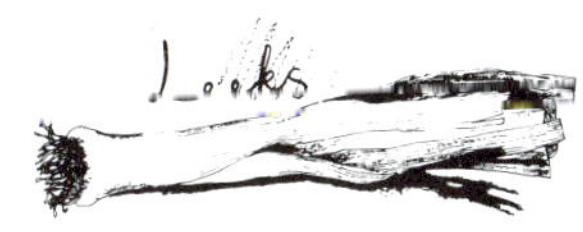

Aubergine & Lentil Bake

Ingredients

2 aubergines, sliced
1 onion
1 or 2 sticks celery, finely chopped
6oz green or brown lentils
Small tin of tomatoes or 1 rounded tablespoon tomato puree
Dried mixed herbs
Pepper and salt

For topping:
¾ pint fairly thick white sauce
2-3oz grated cheese

Method

Put aubergines in a colander, sprinkle well with salt and leave to drain for about half an hour. Fry onion and celery in a little oil until soft. Add lentils, tomatoes, herbs. Cover with about 1½ pints of water, simmer until lentils are tender – about 40 minutes – adding more water if necessary. Drain and pat dry the aubergines; and either fry gently in oil until gold or poach until soft in water. If there is still a lot of water left in the lentil mixture boil rapidly to reduce: the mixture should be moist but not sloppy. Season to taste.

Layer lentil mix and aubergines in a shallow oven-proof dish, finishing with a layer of aubergines. Mix half the cheese into the white sauce and pour it over the top layer of aubergines. Sprinkle the rest of the cheese over the top. Bake 180°C/350°F (gas mark 4) for about 30-40 minutes until golden brown.

Comments

This recipe is immensely variable: you could add carrot, parsnip, mushrooms, red and green peppers for example. Try using fresh tomatoes when they are plentiful, or, instead of herbs, add sweet pickle like Branston or a chutney. You can even use beans instead of lentils.

One of Helen Sharman's favourite dishes – Britain's first astronaut!

HELEN SHARMAN'S MOTHER

Millet & Vegetable Gratinee

Ingredients

4oz millet
1 pint water
3oz butter or margarine
2 medium sized leeks
1 large carrot
4 celery sticks
1oz 100% wholemeal flour
1 pint milk
3 tablespoons chopped parsley
1 teaspoon sage
Grated rind and juice of ½ lemon
Salt and pepper to taste
4oz grated Cheddar cheese

Method

Cook the millet in the measured boiling water until just tender and all the water has been absorbed. Slice the leeks, grate the carrot and finely slice the celery. Melt 2oz butter in a saucepan, add the vegetables and sauté for 10-15 minutes, stirring frequently. Add the millet and stir over very gentle heat to keep warm. Meanwhile, melt the remaining butter in a saucepan. Stir in the flour and cook for 1 minute. Stir in the milk, herbs, lemon rind and juice, and bring to the boil. Reduce heat and simmer for 2 minutes. Pour it over the vegetables and stir well.Adjust seasoning with salt and pepper. Transfer to a warmed serving dish, sprinkle with cheese, and 'bubble' under a hot grill until golden brown.

Serves 4-6.

Comments

The contrasting flavours and textures of millet and vegetables provide a satisfying savoury dish. This is one of my favourite vegetarian dishes. I tend not to tell people what's in it – if you mention 'millet' they assume you're going to dish up bird food! This is a tasty, filling and cheap (or should I say cheep!) recipe and can be made in advance.

HELEN McDERMOTT
Presenter

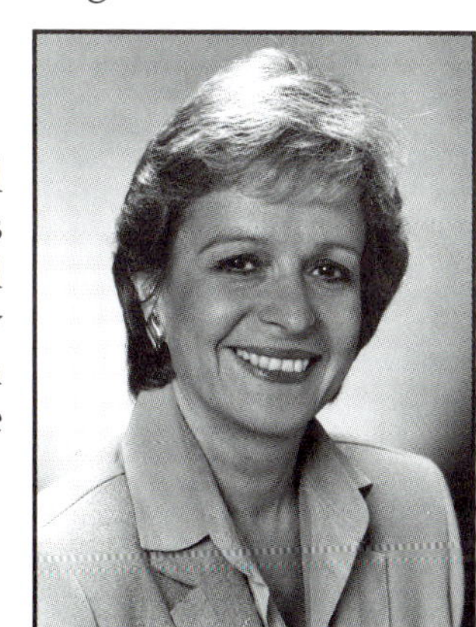

Gratin of Vegetables

Ingredients

8oz celery, sliced
8oz parsnips, peeled and diced
8oz carrots, peeled and diced
8oz onions, peeled and sliced
8oz leeks, cleaned and sliced
8oz mushrooms, washed and sliced
6oz Cheddar cheese, grated
Salt and freshly ground black pepper

Method

Preheat the oven to 200°C/400°F (gas mark 6). Cook all the vegetables except the mushrooms together in boiling water until they are just tender, then drain. Add half the grated cheese and the mushrooms to the vegetables, and some salt and pepper to taste. Spoon the mixture into a shallow oven-proof dish and sprinkle with the remaining cheese. Cook in the oven for about 30 minutes, or until golden brown and crisp on top.

Serves 4. Calories per serving: 260.

R. JAMES
Exeter Branch

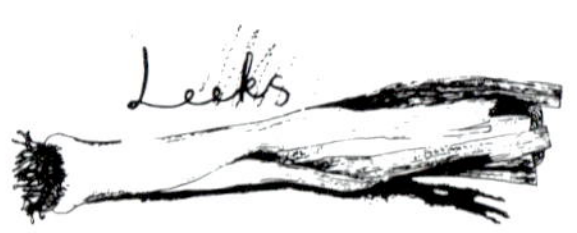

Braised Red Cabbage with Apples

Ingredients

2lb red cabbage
1lb onions, chopped small
1lb cooking apples, peeled, cored and chopped small
3 tablespoons wine vinegar
3 tablespoons brown sugar
1 clove garlic, chopped very small
¼ whole nutmeg freshly grated (2 teaspoons ground nutmeg can be used)
¼ level teaspoon ground cinnamon
¼ level teaspoon ground cloves
½oz butter
Salt and freshly milled black pepper

Method

Preheat oven to 150°C/300°F (gas mark 2). Discard tougher outer leaves of cabbage and cut into quarters and remove hard stalk, then shred cabbage finely. In a fairly large casserole, arrange a layer of shredded cabbage seasoned with salt and pepper, then a layer of chopped onions and apples with a sprinkling of garlic, spices and sugar. Continue with these alternate layers until everything is in. Now pour in the wine vinegar, add a knob of butter. Put lid on casserole. Cook very slowly for 2½-3 hours, stirring everything round once or twice during cooking.

Serves 4.

Comments

Red cabbage, once cooked, will keep warm without coming to any harm. It will also reheat very successfully, so it can be made in advance if necessary. Also it can be frozen in suitable containers for future use. Very good with pork, lamb, sausages, etc.

VI WRIGHT
National Office, Alzheimer's Disease Society, Balham

Savoury Tofu

Ingredients

1 large chopped Spanish onion
1 chopped clove garlic
2 tablespoons vegetable oil
3 medium-sized sticks celery, chopped
1 packet plain tofu (just under 1lb)
4oz oatmeal
3 chopped tomatoes
3 tablespoons soy sauce (tamari is good)
3 tablespoons tomato puree
¼ teaspoon cayenne pepper
1 teaspoon dry mustard powder
1 teaspoon chopped basil
2 tablespoons chopped fresh parsley
Ground black pepper
Ground sea salt

Method

Put the chopped Spanish onion into a big mixing bowl. Add all the other ingredients and mix together. Scoop into large pyrex. Microwave on high for 10-15 minutes; or in oven at 180°C/350°F (gas mark 4) for an hour covered with foil.

PAULETTE MICKLEWOOD
Oxfordshire Branch

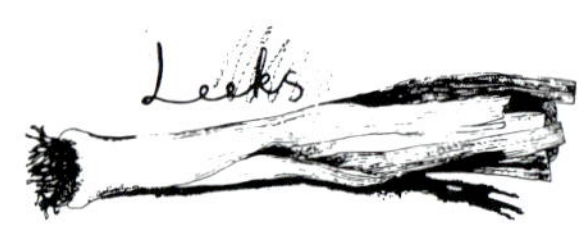

Cheddar Curry

Ingredients

1oz butter or margarine
1 onion, chopped
1oz plain flour
1 or 2 teaspoons curry powder, according to taste
½ pint stock
2 level tablespoons sweet chutney
1oz sultanas
6oz cubed Cheddar cheese
4oz long grain rice, cooked
Salt and pepper to taste

Method

Fry onion in a saucepan in butter until golden brown. Add flour and curry powder and stir over a gentle heat. Gradually blend in the stock and continue to heat and whisk until the sauce thickens. Add salt, pepper, chutney, sultanas and cheese and mix well. Serve hot on a plate with cooked rice.

Comments

This is a quick standby recipe using things normally found in the store cupboard.

BELLE CHALDICOTT

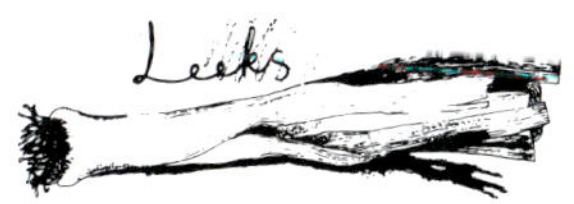

Leek & Mushroom Pie

Ingredients

For wholemeal shortcrust pastry:
12oz 100% wholemeal flour
6oz fat

Beaten egg to glaze

For filling:
2½oz butter or margarine
1½lb leeks, trimmed and sliced
1lb open cap mushrooms
4 teaspoons 100% wholemeal flour
1 vegetable stock cube
2 garlic cloves, crushed
Ground nutmeg to taste
Salt and pepper
4 tablespoons chopped parsley
7oz low fat skimmed milk cheese
2 eggs, lightly beaten

Method

Preparation time: 35 minutes. Cooking time: 30-40 minutes.

Melt 2 oz butter/margarine in pan, add leeks and cook until tender. Remove leeks and reserve juices. Add mushrooms and cook until tender. Drain mushrooms and add to leeks. Put reserved juices into a jug and, if necessary, make up to ¼ pint with stock. Melt remaining butter, stir in flour and cook for 1 minute. Add reserved liquid, stock cube, garlic, nutmeg, salt and pepper. Stir over heat until sauce boils and thickens. Simmer gently to thicken. Combine mushrooms, leeks and sauce and stir in the parsley, cheese and beaten egg. Cool. Make and roll out pastry to line a 9″ pie plate. Put the cold mushroom and leek mixture into the pastry case and brush edges with beaten egg. Roll out remaining pastry to cover pie. Seal and trim edges. Cut a small hole in top of pie. Brush with beaten egg. Bake at 200°C/400°F (gas mark 6) for 30-40 minutes. Serves 8.

MARY CALLAND
Rhyl and District Branch

Spinach Pots

Ingredients

8oz frozen chopped leaf spinach (not puree)
1 medium onion, finely chopped
1 large or 2 small cloves garlic, finely chopped
2 tablespoons cottage cheese
2 tablespoons plain yoghurt
1 tablespoon chopped parsley
1 tablespoon lemon juice
2 hard boiled eggs
Salt and pepper to taste
Grated carrot

Method

Cook the spinach according to the instructions on the packet. You can use fresh spinach and then chop it and cook it for not more than 10 minutes in very little water. When the spinach is nearly cooked add the onion, garlic, parsley and seasonings. In another bowl mix together the cottage cheese, yoghurt, lemon juice and 1½ chopped hard boiled eggs, saving some of the yolk and white for the garnish. Strain the spinach mixture particularly well and allow to cool. Blend the contents of the two bowls together and put into ramekins. Garnish with the separated chopped egg white and yolk and top with grated carrot.

Comments

Serve with a night-cap of chilled Muscadet!

One of the most miserable sides of the House of Commons is the fact that the hours are quite ridiculous. Enjoying my wife's cooking is therefore a rare treat, reserved only for Sundays. One night, however, after a 2am finish I got home to find these delicious Spinach Pots waiting for me in the fridge. These are now a regular feature of late night sittings, and I almost look forward to them. They're thoroughly healthy too!

JEREMY HANLEY, MP
Parliamentary Under Secretary of State in the Northern Ireland Office; Minister for Health and Personal Social Services; Minister for Agriculture and Rural Development

Savoury Spaghetti

Ingredients

4oz spaghetti (or macaroni)
4oz cheese
1lb tomatoes
½ pint stock
½oz cornflour
Pinch of mixed herbs
1 onion
1oz butter
Seasoning

Method

Grease pie dish. Wipe tomatoes and slice. Peel and slice onion. Melt butter in saucepan. Add tomatoes and onion. Cook for a few minutes; add stock and herbs. Bring to boil, season well. Simmer until tender. Cook spaghetti in boiling salted water until tender, and drain. Grate cheese finely. Rub tomato sauce through sieve. Return puree to saucepan. Thicken with cornflour and a little water. Bring to boil and stir for a few minutes. Layer cheese, spaghetti, tomato and cheese. Cook in oven, then brown under grill.

VEENA JACKSON
Nottingham Branch

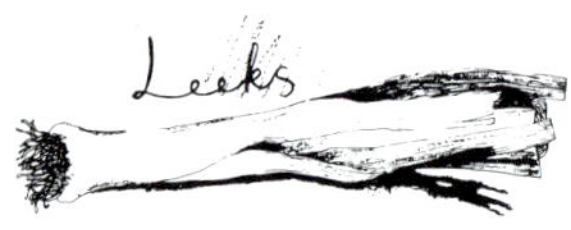

Mushroom & Tomato Savoury

Ingredients

8oz soft breadcrumbs
4oz milled nuts
4oz margarine
8oz mushrooms
8oz tomatoes
Salt and pepper
1 teaspoon marjoram

Method

Fry breadcrumbs and nuts in 3 oz margarine until golden. Fry washed and chopped mushrooms and tomatoes in rest of fat. Grease oven-proof dish; fill alternate layers of the two mixtures, seasoning each layer. The top layer should be the crumb mixture. Cook for 30 minutes at 190°C/375°F (gas mark 5).

DAWN MARRIOTT
Camden Branch

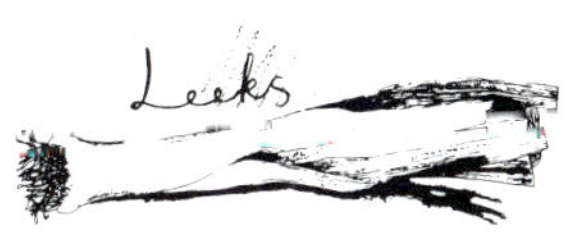

Very Low Fat Chips & Roast Potatoes

Method

Peel potatoes and slice as if for chips. Place in appropriate container for use in microwave oven with about two tablespoons water. Cook on high for about five minutes or until soft enough to probe with a fork.

Brush with oil and place under medium grill, turning as required, for about 10 minutes.

W. G. HOPCRAFT
Seaton

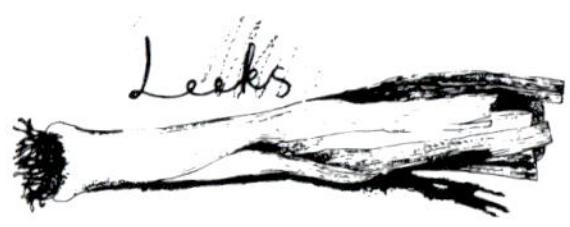

Redeemed Swede

Ingredients

1 swede
1 lemon
Some parsley
2oz butter

Food processor or blender
Saucepan
Sharp knife

Method

Boil swede until soft. In a food processor, place 2oz butter and 2 or 3 heads of parsley, and the juice and thin outer peel of a lemon. Blend on the fast speed for two seconds or so. Add the softened swede with a little of the water it was boiled in. Process on the fast speed for a few seconds until pureed. Turn out into a vegetable dish. Sprinkle with chopped parsley.

Serves 3 or 4.

DAVID SHEPPARD
The Right Reverend Bishop of Liverpool

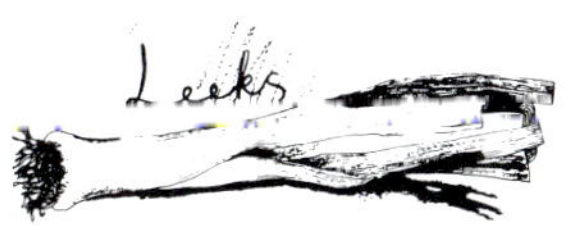

Vegetable Delight

Ingredients

1 onion, chopped
1 tablespoon oil
1 small tin red kidney beans
1 small tin butter beans
1 small tin chopped tomatoes
4 mushrooms, chopped
1 courgette, chopped
Salt and pepper
½-1 teaspoon chilli powder

Method

Fry onion, add all the other ingredients and cook for approx 10 minutes.

Comments

Good, Quick and Healthy!

CHRISTINE ELSTON
Hull and East Yorkshire Branch

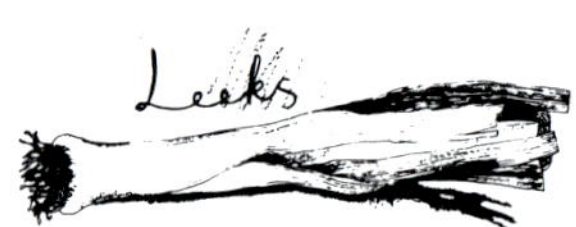

Puds

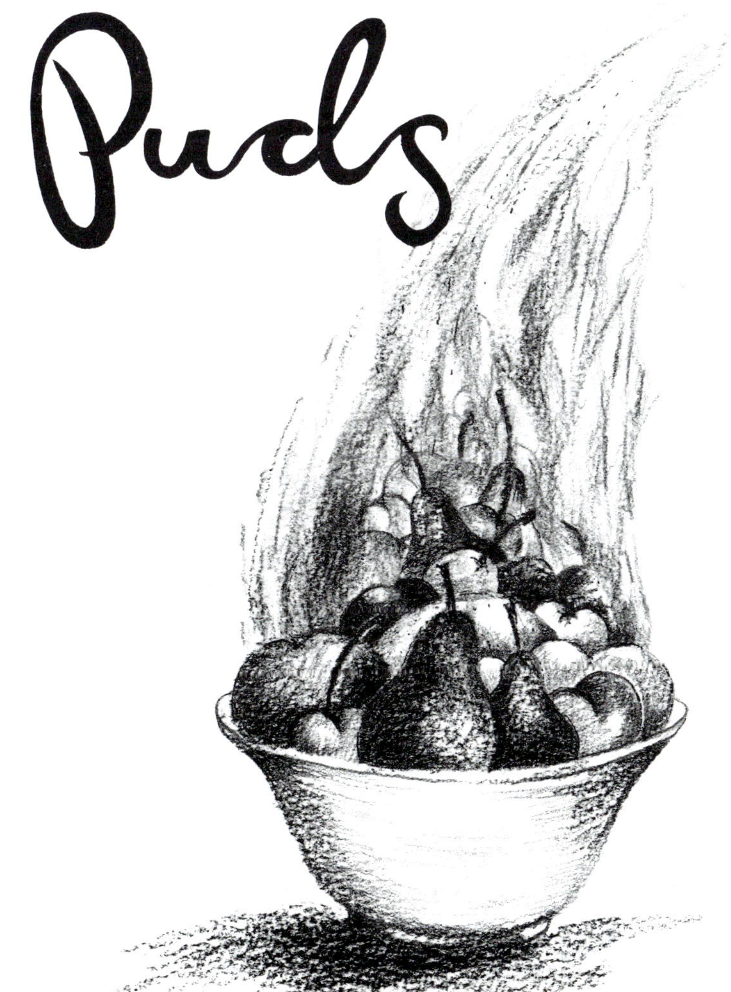

Orange & Lemon Flan

Ingredients

For the filling:

2 eggs
3oz caster sugar
4fl oz single cream
4oz stale cake crumbs
Grated zest and juice of 1 small orange
Few drops of almond essence

For the topping:

2 large thin-skinned lemons
2 small thin-skinned oranges
5fl oz water
3oz sugar
4 tablespoons sieved marmalade or orange jelly

Method

Preparation and cooking time: 1 hour.

Heat the oven to 190°C/375°F (gas mark 5).

Prepare the filling by whisking the eggs with sugar until thick and creamy. Add the remaining ingredients and beat vigorously until well mixed. Spread the mixture in the flan shell and bake for 30-40 minutes or until well risen, golden and firm to touch in the centre.

Meanwhile, prepare the topping by slicing the oranges and lemons very thinly, removing all the pips. If the pith is thick, peel the fruit with a sharp knife, as you would apples, or they may be rather bitter. Dissolve the sugar in the water in a shallow, wide pan and bring to the boil. Lay the orange and lemon slices in the syrup and simmer for 3 minutes, then remove and drain well. Boil the remaining

continued

Orange & Lemon Flan (cont.)

Method (cont.)

syrup until reduced by half. Stir in the marmalade and heat until it is completely melted to give a good, rich glaze.

Arrange the orange and lemon slices on top of the flan and brush generously with the glaze. Place under a hot grill (broiler) for a few minutes until the glaze is bubbling and caramelised.

Serve warm or cold, decorated with pieces of glacé cherries if wished, and an accompanying jug of cream.

Serves 6-8.

THE RT. HON. MARGARET THATCHER, FRS, MP

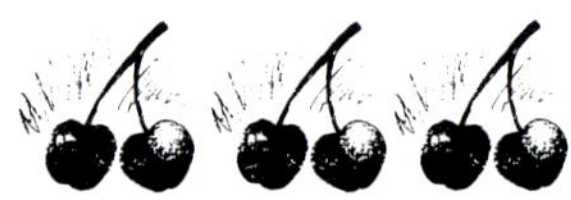

Christmas Trifle

Ingredients

4 slices of Christmas pudding
Grated rind and juice of 1 orange
2 tablespoons custard powder
2oz sugar
1 pint milk
5fl oz fresh orange, concentrated
1 tablespoon brandy
1oz flaked almonds, roasted

Method

Cut pudding into small pieces and place in base of serving dish. Sprinkle with orange juice. Blend together the custard powder, 1oz sugar and 2 tablespoons of milk. Bring remaining milk to boil. Pour into blended custard. Return to heat stirring continuously until it boils and thickens. Allow to cool and pour over the Christmas pudding. Whip cream, mix in orange rind, brandy, remaining sugar. Spread cream mixture over custard. Sprinkle with toasted almonds.

Serves 6.

MRS G. MERRITT

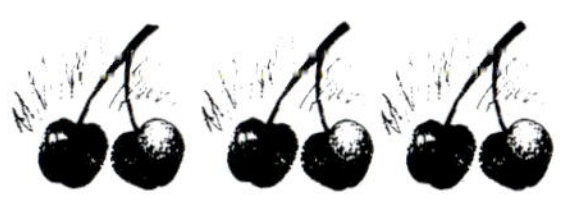

Wiltshire Pudding

Ingredients

3 well beaten eggs
1 pint milk
Flour
Salt
1 cup redcurrants
½ cup raspberries
Butter
Brown sugar
Pudding sauce

Method

Mix well: 3 well-beaten eggs, a pint of milk and as much flour as will make a thick batter, and a little salt. Beat it for some minutes, then stir in gently a large cupful of redcurrants and half their quantity of raspberries. Boil in cloth for two hours.

Turn the pudding out on the dish it is to be served on. Cut into slices about ¾″ thick, but do not separate them. Put a thin slice of butter and some brown sugar between the layers and serve with pudding sauce in a tureen.

Comments

You may make this pudding without raspberries.

MARLBOROUGH & DISTRICT CARERS GROUP

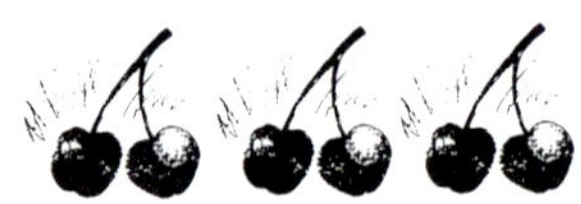

Warsfell Peach Dessert

Ingredients

7 whole peaches
2 tablespoons sugar
2oz butter
1 beaten egg yolk
5 almond macaroons (approx), crumbled

Method

Puree and mash one whole peach. Add 1oz sugar, butter, egg yolk and crumbled macaroons to the pureed peach. Mix well. Fill each peach half with some of the mixture piling it up in the middle. Arrange peaches in fire-proof dish and dot with remaining butter. Bake in a moderate oven. Serve hot or cold with cream. Serves 6.

MRS B. M. PURDUE
Buckhurst Hill, Essex

Gooseberry Pie

Comments

Although I do not know the recipe, I am very fond of Gooseberry Pie with Custard. The custard complements the bitterness of the gooseberry.

RUSS ABBOTT
Entertainer

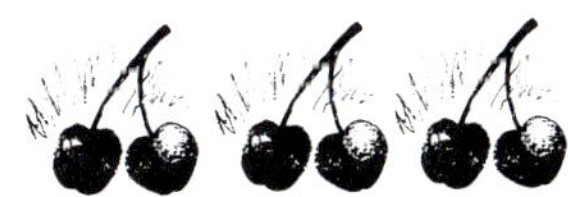

Lemon Fridge Cake

Ingredients

1 packet trifle sponges
4oz butter
6oz caster sugar
3 eggs separated
Grated rind and juice of 2 lemons
5oz carton whipping cream
4 thin slices lemon
Grated plain chocolate (optional)

Method

Line sides and base of 2lb loaf tin with foil overlapped at rim. Cut sponges into 3 thin pieces and line base and sides of tin, reserving pieces leftover. Beat butter and sugar until fluffy, beat in egg yolks, then beat in juice and rind slowly – don't worry if it curdles. Stiffly beat egg whites and fold into lemon mixture. Place half in lined tin, cover with sponges, then repeat layers. Fold foil over to cover sponges and chill in fridge overnight. Remove foil from top and invert cake on to plate. Remove rest of foil and decorate with cream, chocolate and lemon slices.

MRS BETTY BUCKLEY
Occupational Therapy Technician, Thameside General Hospital

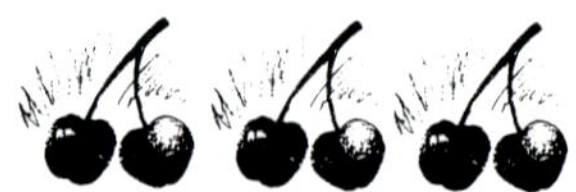

Mixed Fruit Flambe

Ingredients

2 medium nectarines
4oz cherries
1 medium banana
½ medium firm papaya
4fl oz water
Grated zest of ½ lemon
5 teaspoons sugar
1 teaspoon arrowroot
1 teaspoon water
6 tablespoons kirsch or rum

Method

Halve the nectarines, remove the stones and cut each nectarine half into four wedges. Stone the cherries, slice the banana diagonally into thick slices. Scoop the seeds out of the papaya, peel and dice. Place all the fruit, water and lemon zest in a saucepan, cover and simmer for about 10 minutes until the fruit is just cooked. Stir in the sugar and remove from the heat. Remove the fruit. Blend the arrowroot with the water, stir into the syrup, bring to the boil, simmer for 1 minute, stirring all the time. Replace the fruit, stir gently over a low heat, add the kirsch or rum, set alight and serve immediately.

MALLING CARERS' SUPPORT GROUP

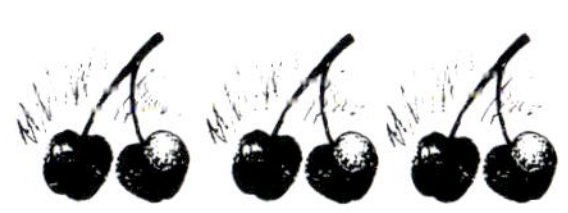

Guards' Pudding

Ingredients

6oz fresh white breadcrumbs
6oz chopped shredded suet
or butter
4oz brown or sand sugar
3 tablespoons strawberry jam
1 large or 2 small eggs
1 level teaspoon bicarbonate of soda
Pinch of salt

For the sauce:
1 whole egg
1 egg yolk
1½oz caster sugar
1 large tablespoon orange juice

Method

Mix dry ingredients together. Add jam and egg beaten up with bicarbonate of soda. Mix thoroughly and then turn into a well greased mould which should be a little more than 3 parts full. Steam for 4 hours.

Sauce:
Place sauce ingredients in a bowl and then place in a further bowl of very hot water. Whisk until thick and frothy. Serve immediately with pudding. If not, whisk for one minute before serving.

Comments

This is my favourite pudding.

BRIAN JOHNSTON
Cricket Commentator

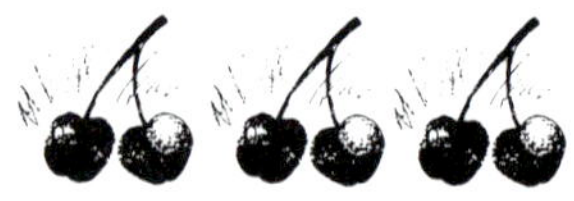

Fruit Sponge

Ingredients

1 banana, peeled and sliced
6oz fresh prepared pineapple, cut into small chunks, or drained tinned pineapple chunks
4-6oz sliced tinned peaches, drained and cut into chucks – reserve juice
Pinch ground cloves

For sponge:
4oz flour (mixture of white, brown and wholemeal)
1 teaspoon baking powder, if using plain flour
2oz soft margarine
2oz caster or soft brown sugar
1 tablespoon fruit syrup
1 egg, size 3

Method

Prepare oven at 200°C/400°F (gas mark 6). Place fruit in 2 pint oven dish and mix. Sprinkle cloves over fruit. Mix sponge ingredients together to a smooth and spoon-dropping consistency and spread over fruit. Place in oven (middle shelf) and cook for 30 minutes until brown, risen and firm. Serve hot or cold with cream or custard. Serves 4.

Comments

This sponge is ideal for using "odds and ends" of fresh or tinned fruit. Numerous combinations can be used with a variety of different spices depending on choice and availability. This is one example only. Add sugar if the fruit is really sharp.

If there are only two of you, resist the temptation to be greedy and keep half the pudding for the next day – eat it either cold or warm it up in the oven after you have finished cooking the main course and turned the oven off.

MRS J. E. WILLIAMS
Mid-Sussex Branch

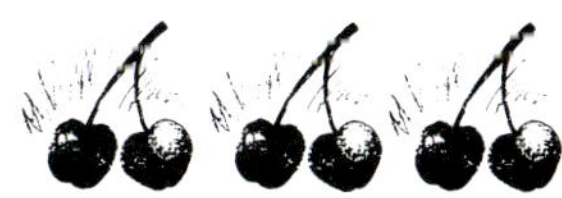

Slimmers' Ice Cream

Ingredients

4 eggs
4oz caster sugar
½ pint double or whipping cream
Strawberries/raspberries
Drinking chocoloate/vanilla essence

Method

Whisk 4 egg whites and 4oz caster sugar, slowly. (My own recipe says "caster sugar, Eric". Took me an age to decipher that – "little by little", of course!)

Whip ½ pint whipping (or double) cream and bung it in. Add what you fancy. (No, not Guinness.) Vanilla essence, pureed going-soft strawberries or raspberries – my own preference is 2 tablespoons of drinking chocolate and 2 dessertspoons of instant coffee melted in the very minimum of milk. Sharp fruit may need a little icing sugar. (I have also tried small-chopped cherries.)

Freeze it, but remember to remove about 20 minutes before you want to eat it, as it sets like concrete.

PHIL DAY
Norwich

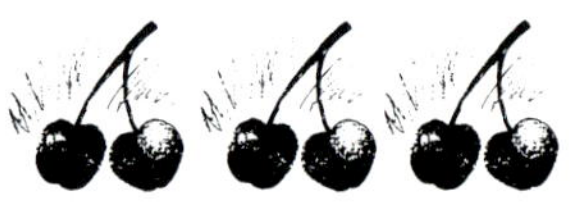

Profiteroles
(WITH HOT CHOCOLATE SAUCE)

Ingredients

For the sauce:
8oz Cadbury's Milk Chocolate
½oz butter
2 tablespoons water
2 level tablespoons Golden Syrup
1 teaspoon vanilla essence

For the profiteroles:
2½oz plain flour, sieved
2oz butter, cut up
1 level teaspoon sugar
5fl oz cold water
2 large eggs, beaten
½ pint double cream, whipped thick for filling

Method

Pre-heat the oven to 215°C/425°F (gas mark 7). Grease a large tray. Put the sugar, water and butter in a pan. Bring to the boil. Tip in the sieved flour all at once then take the pan off the heat and beat until the mixture leaves the side of the pan. Beat in the eggs and make 20 small bun shapes, or use 20 teaspoons of the mixture. Bake for 10 minutes. Reduce the oven temperature to 165°C/325°F (gas mark 3) and bake for another 15 or 20 minutes.

While they are baking, boil a saucepan of water and put a sieve on the top of the pan. Put the chocolate into a bowl in the sieve to melt, then add the butter, water, syrup and vanilla essence and stir in well.

Cool the profiteroles on a wire rack and when you are ready to serve, split them a little. Put the cream in with a teaspoon and pour the chocolate over and serve.

BONNIE TYLER

Impossible Custard Tart

Ingredients

4 eggs
3oz butter
½ cup plain flour
2 cups milk
1 cup sugar
1 cup coconut
1 teaspoon vanilla essence

Method

Mix all ingredients in a blender. (I used half the quantity in a blender, but a food processor is better for the full quantity.) Pour mixture into a greased 9″ pie plate. Bake at 180°C/350°F (gas mark 4) for one hour, or until set.

The flour settles and makes a crust base, coconut forms the topping, and egg custard filling forms the centre.

Comments

I collected this recipe while on holiday "down-under" in Adelaide; it is easy and a great time-saver. Our hostess commented: "You realise, of course, when we do these recipes we're standing on our heads. Think how much easier it will be for you standing on your feet!!!"

OLIVE ROWETT
Lewisham Branch

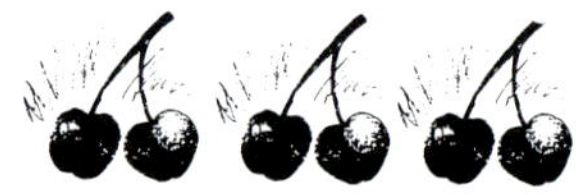

Cheesecake Tart

Ingredients

For pastry:
6oz plain flour
3oz butter
1 teaspoon sugar
Milk to mix

For filling:
2 oz butter
3oz sugar
3 eggs, separated
2oz ground almonds
1oz fine semolina
8oz cream cheese
Grated rind and juice of 1 lemon
2oz raisins, stoned

Method

Rub the fat into the flour, add the sugar and enough milk to make a firm dough. Knead lightly. Line one 8″ sandwich tin with the pastry.

Cream the butter and the sugar together for the filling. Add the egg yolks, almonds, semolina, cheese, lemon rind and juice and raisins. Mix well. Beat egg whites until stiff and fold into mixture with a metal spoon.

Pour into pastry case. Bake in the centre of a moderate oven for 50 minutes or until filling is set.

W. BARTLETT
Buckinghamshire Branch

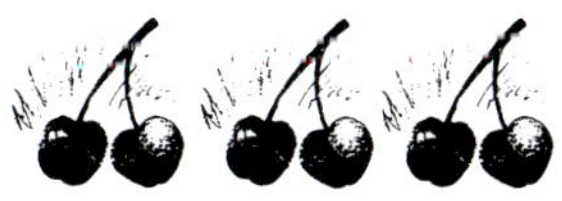

Parfait au Marron

Ingredients

4oz bitter cooking chocolate
3oz caster sugar
2½fl oz water
1lb tin unsweetened chestnut puree
2 eggs
6oz softened butter
Whipped cream
Chocolate vermicelli

Method

Break the chocolate into pieces, and put it in a saucepan with the sugar and water. Stir it over a gentle heat until the chocolate and sugar have melted. Leave to cool slightly, then mix it into the chestnut puree.

Separate the eggs and beat the yolks into the mixture, one at a time. Cut the butter into pieces, and beat them in – an electric mixer makes this stage much easier. Whisk the egg whites until they are stiff, then fold them into the mixture.

Butter in 1¾ pint mould, or two small ones and fill with the mixture. Cover and place in the fridge until the following day.

Turn the parfait out of its mould and serve it with whipped cream, decorated with chocolate vermicelli.

DUNCAN KYLE

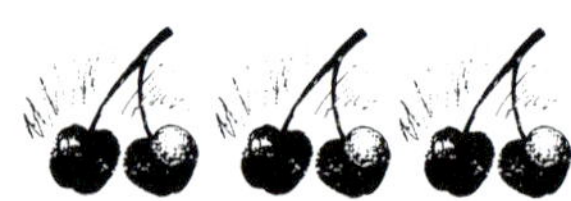

Himmel Fritter

Ingredients

2 eggs, well-beaten
1 cup sugar
2 heaped tablespoons flour
1 teaspoon baking powder
8oz dates
8oz walnuts
Oranges
Bananas
½ pint double or whipping cream

Method

Mix all ingredients together except oranges, bananas and cream and bake in greased baking tin for 30 minutes or until light and brown. Cool and break up for base. Cover pieces thickly with sliced oranges and bananas. Top with ½ pint of whipped cream.

Comments

M. .m. .mmm. . .!!

MEG SKINNER
National Office, Alzheimer's Disease Society, Balham

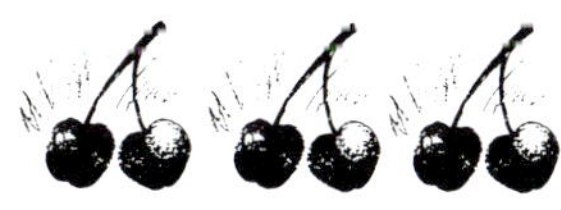

Chestnut 'Stockade' Pudding

Ingredients

About 35 boudoir biscuits
A little milk
1lb tin sweetened chestnut puree (or use unsweetend puree, and sweeten to taste)
3oz unsalted butter
Dessertspoon (or more) rum or brandy
½ pint stiffly whipped double cream

Method

Grease a small round cake tin with removable bottom. Break ½″ off boudoir biscuits, dip the broken ends in the milk and line the sides of the tin. Use the broken off bits (and extra biscuits as necessary) to line the bottom. Soften the butter, add the chestnut puree and rum or brandy, and mix well. Pour this into the mould. Cover with the whipped cream into which a little more brandy/rum has been stirred. Cool in refrigerator overnight, or longer.

Comments

Delicious – very rich!

DAWN MARRIOTT
Camden Branch

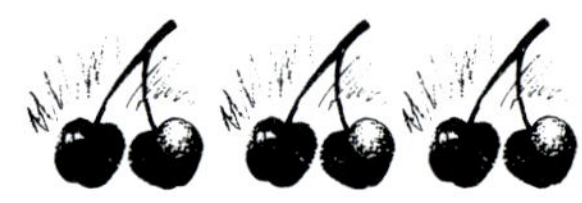

Christmas Pudding

Ingredients

1½lb seedless raisins
8oz currants
4oz glace cherries
8oz mixed peel
12oz fine breadcrumbs
8 eggs
1 teaspoon each of nutmeg, cinnamon and allspice
4oz blanched almonds
12oz chopped suet
¼ pint brown ale or stout
6 tablespoons brandy or rum

Method

Makes one 2 pint and one 1½ pint pudding.

Line basins with greased paper, and scald pudding cloths. Prepare dried fruit, rub in some flour, then shake. Add peel, cherries and almonds. Mix fruit with suet and crumbs, add nutmeg, cinnamon and allspice. Beat the eggs, stir into dry ingredients, then add rum and beer to dropping consistency. Fill bowls ¾ full, steam/boil 2 pint for 7-8 hours, 1½ pint for 6 hours. (Divide boiling time between day of making and day of eating.)

Serve with brandy butter, brandy cream or white or custard sauce or a combination.

Comments

This is my "no-flour, no-sugar" Christmas Pudding – the yummy sweetness comes from the fruit and the rich, dark colour from long boiling.

LORNA S. RAYNER

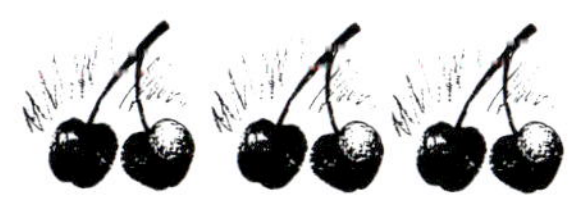

John Peel Tart

Ingredients

8oz shortcrust pastry
1oz chopped peel
1oz margarine
½ teaspoon spice
6oz cleaned currants
4oz golden syrup
1oz ground almonds
2 teaspoon lemon juice

Method

Warm margarine and syrup together. When melted stir in all the other filling ingredients. Allow to cool. Line 7″ pie plate with half pastry and fill with filling. Cover with remaining pastry, sealing edges. Bake for 40 minutes at 200°-210°C/ 400°-425°F (gas mark 6-7). Serve warm or cold.

PENRITH SUPPORT GROUP

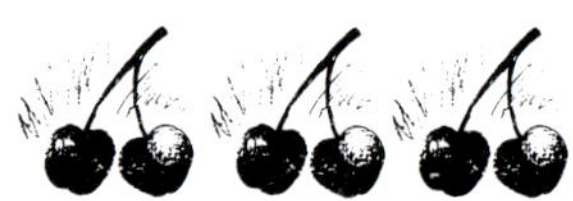

Apricot Almond Bake

Ingredients

For base:

15oz medium tin apricot halves (drained)

2 tins apricot pie filling

For topping:

8oz white sugar

6oz soft margarine (Flora)

6oz ground almonds

Few drops of almond essence

2 eggs

Method

Chop up apricot halves and put with pie filling into 1½ pint souffle dish. Beat together all ingredients for topping and spread over fruit. Bake in low/moderate oven for about 45 minutes.

Serves 6.

Comments

This is an easy "no-fail" pudding. It can be made the previous day and left over in the fridge. Delicious with lashings of plain ice cream, but loaded with calories!

For smaller families use half the topping and one tin of filling with tin of apricots.

MARJORIE STONE
Vice Chairman, Alzheimer's Disease Society

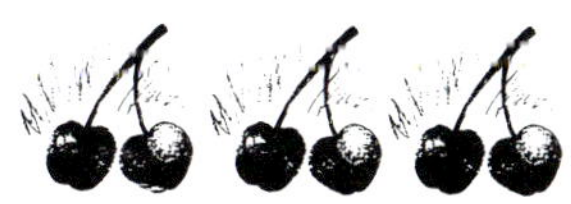

Pumpkin Pie

Ingredients

8oz shortcrust pastry

For filling:
Chopped stem ginger to taste
8oz mashed cooked pumpkin
4oz soft brown sugar
1 tablespoon thick honey
Grated rind and juice of 1 lemon
Grated rind and juice of 1 orange
2 eggs, well-beaten

To finish:
¼ pint double cream
1 teaspoon caster sugar
¼ teaspoon nutmeg
2oz walnuts (chopped roughly) or flaked toasted almonds

Method

Set oven at 180°C/350°F (gas mark 4). Line the dish with pastry and place ginger on the bottom.

For the filling:
Mix the sugar, honey and the grated fruit rinds, then stir in the mashed pumpkin. Mix with the rest of the filling ingredients. Pour the mixture into the prepared pastry case and bake for 45-55 minutes, or until a knife inserted in the filling comes out clean. Allow to cool.

To finish:
Whip the cream, sweeten with the sugar and add the nutmeg. Just before serving, cover the pie with cream and sprinkle with the chopped nuts.

THE RT. HON. EDWARD HEATH, MBE, MP

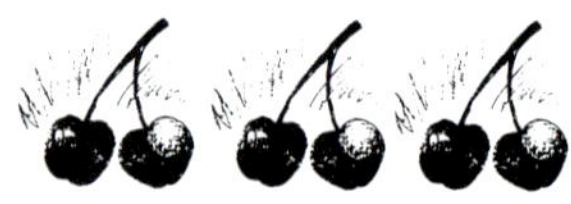

The Only Pudding

Ingredients

½ pint double cream, stiffly whipped
½ pint yoghurt (the thick Greek kind is best, but any plain yoghurt will do)
A little sugar
Fruit – fresh or tinned or a mixture of both – drained of any juice or syrup

Method

Mix the cream and yoghurt together Chop the fruit and fold it in, and add sugar to taste. Put a little fruit on top for decoration and serve with shortbread fingers or crisp biscuits such as 'lanques de chat'. You can vary the proportion of fruit and the kind of fruit. It works well with strawberries, raspberries, fresh apples and pears, dried fruit or mincemeat. Recently I used a jar of blackcurrants (with the juice drained off) and served Waitrose blackcurrant sorbet with it – superb! You can also vary the proportion of cream and yoghurt to make it more or less rich. Serves 6.

Comments

This is almost the only pudding I ever make nowadays, because it is quick, easy and delicious, can be made in advance or at the last minute, and is capable of endless variations.

LADY NAIRNE
Chipping Norton, Oxon.

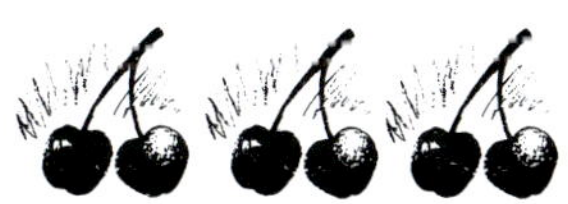

Indian Ice Cream – Kulfi

Ingredients

1 small tin condensed milk
5oz carton single cream
14oz tin evaporated milk
2 tablespoons rose water or 1 teaspoon almond essence or 1 teaspoon vanilla essence
½ cup icing sugar
2 tablespoons ground almonds
1 tablespoon whole pistachio nuts
1 tablespoon sliced pistachio nuts
1 teaspoon green colouring

Method

Mix all the ingredients well. Pour into ice cream moulds or ice trays. Cover with grease-proof paper and put into the freezer.

Comments

Warning: This recipe is not for the fainthearted! Definitely not for slimmers! Only share this with your best friends!

JOHN MARLOW

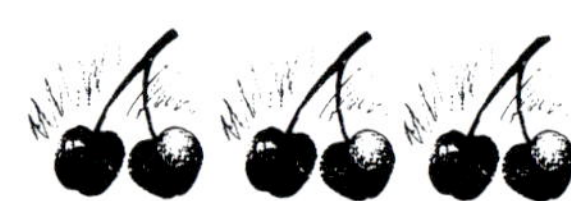

Stuffed Pears in Cointreau

Ingredients

7oz sugar
¾ pint water
Thinly pared rind of 2 oranges, shredded and blanched
Juice of 2 oranges
6 William pears
1-2 tablespoons Cointreau

For filling:
3oz ground almonds
2oz icing sugar
1oz softened butter
Grated rind and juice of 1 lemon and 1 orange

Method

Bring the sugar, water and orange shreds to the boil and cook for 5 minutes until a syrup forms. Add the orange juice. Mix together the almonds, sugar, butter and lemon and orange rinds. Bind with a little orange juice if necessary. Peel the pears leaving them whole, then remove the core. Dip in lemon juice and fill with almond mixture. Stand in an oven-proof dish and pour the syrup over with any remaining orange and lemon juice. Cover and bake in a moderate oven 180°C/350°F (gas mark 4) for 20-25 minutes, until tender. Baste with syrup during cooking. Remove pears to a serving dish and keep warm. Boil the syrup until reduced. Add liquor and spoon over pears.

Serves 6.

MR CHATER
Hon. Secretary
Colchester Stanway Townswomen's Guild, Great Chippendale

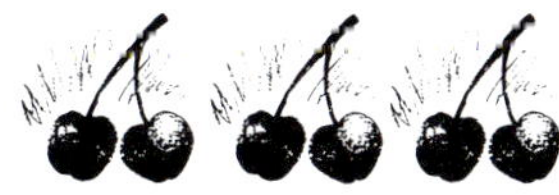

Chocolate & Mint Matchmaker Ice

Ingredients

7oz dark chocolate
3 tablespoons cocoa powder
½ teaspoon powdered coffee
17fl oz whipping cream
4 fl oz milk
2 whole eggs
3 egg yolks
2 tablespoons honey
1 teaspoon natural vanilla essence
3oz 'Mint Matchmaker' – roughly broken

Method

Mix cocoa and coffee powder to a paste with the milk in a heavy-based pan. Break up the chocolate and add to the pan with ½ pint of the cream. Heat gently until the chcolate melts. Stir until smooth, and brought to boiling point. Meanwhile, beat eggs, yolks and honey for 1 minute until thick and pale. Gradually add the boiling chocolate mixture, beating all the time. Beat for a further 30 seconds. Stir in remaining cream. Cool. Add chopped Matchmakers and turn into ice-cream machine (or into tin-foil containers for the deep freeze – but keep stirring whilst freezing).

LADY MARTHA PONSONBY
Oxford

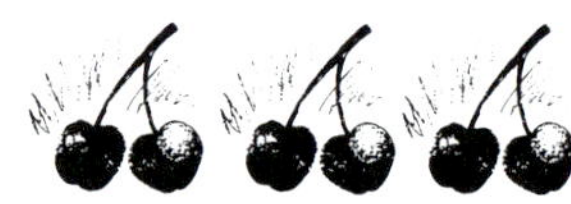

Apple Crumble

Ingredients

1½lb Bramley apples
4oz brown sugar
A little grated lemon rind
½ gill water (approx)
3oz butter or margarine
6oz plain flour
3oz caster sugar
½ teaspoon ground ginger

Method

Peel, core and slice the apples into a pan. Add water, sugar and lemon rind. Cook gently with lid on pan until soft. Place in a greased 2 pint pie dish. Rub the fat into the flour until the consistency of fine breadcrumbs. Add the caster sugar, ground ginger and mix well. Sprinkle the crumble over the apple; press down lightly. Bake in a moderate oven 180°C/350°F (gas mark 4) until golden brown, and the apples are cooked – about 30-40 minutes depending on the cooking quality of apples. Dredge with caster sugar and serve with custard or cream.

Serves 6.

Comments

The reason why I like Apple Crumble is because I love Bramley apples – they remind me of my Mum. She always put some on top of the wardrobe rubbed with vaseline for apple sauce for the turkey or capon at Christmas.

DORA BRYAN
Actress

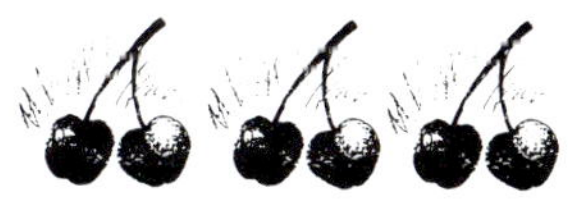

Microwave Steamed Pudding

Ingredients

1 tablespoon butter or margarine, melted
2 tablespoons brown sugar
¼ cup grated carrot
1 teaspoon ground ginger
5 tablespoons flour
¼ teaspoon bicarbonate of soda
1 tablespoon milk (enough to make a soft mix)

Method

Mix all the ingredients together. Grease a large cup – put mixture in. Microwave on HIGH for 90 seconds. Leave to stand for 2 minutes before unmoulding.

Comments

For 2 in a hurry!

GRACE DU FAUR
ADARDS

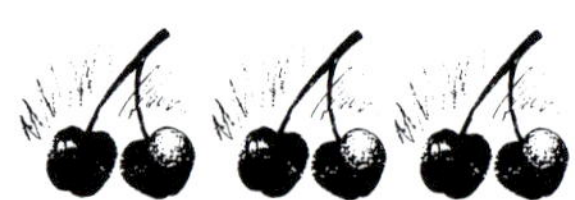

Dominica Banana Trifle

Ingredients

1 Madeira cake
1 pint milk
2 bananas
2 eggs plus 2 egg yolks
2 tablespoons caster sugar
10fl oz double cream

Method

Bring the milk to the boil in a saucepan. Beat together the eggs, egg yolks and sugar and strain on to milk. Cook gently, without boiling, stirring until the custard thickens slightly.

Crumble the Madeira cake into the bottom of the trifle dish. Slice the bananas and layer on top of the cake crumbs. Pour over the cold custard. Lightly whip cream. Top the custard with half the cream and pipe the remainder on top and decorate. Further decorate with paper parasols, crisp wafers, nuts and sliced bananas and cherries.

RICHARD WOLD
Marathon Runner

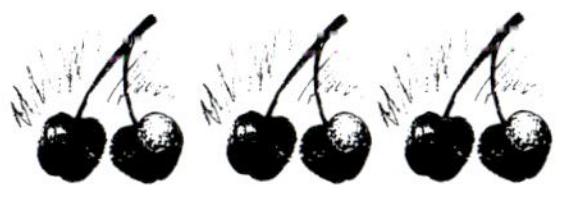

Roly Poly Pudding

Ingredients

8oz self-raising flour
3oz butter
1oz caster sugar

4 tablespoons milk
Pinch of salt

For filling:
Jam or fruit

3 tablespoons water

Method

Sieve flour and salt together. Rub in butter, add sugar, mix to a soft dough with the milk. Roll out pastry to a rectangle, approx. 12″ × 10″. Cover with jam or fruit. Moisten edges of dough with water, then roll as for Swiss roll. Press joins gently together. Lift into dish. Make 2 slits on top, brush with milk. Pour 3 tablespoons of water into dish. Bake in a hot oven for 15 minutes then reduce to moderate oven for rest of time (45 minutes in all).

Comments

While cooking, tap dance round the kitchen – good for the figure. At Christmas, dress your Roly Poly Pudding in silver paper, ribbon and tinsel to look like a Christmas Cracker.

THE ROLY POLYS
Entertainers

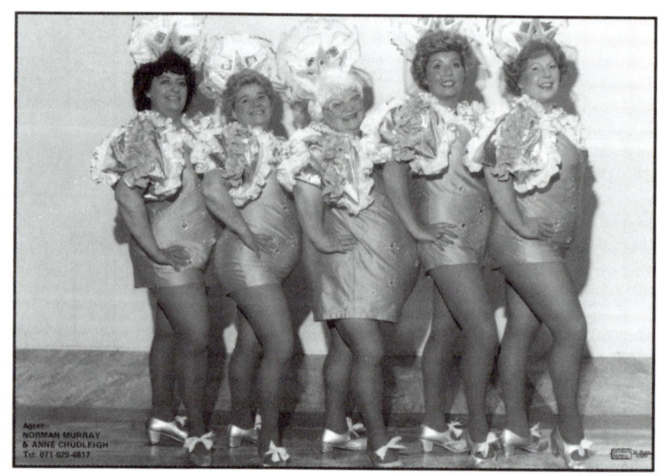

Pavlova
(THE NEW ZEALAND WAY)

Ingredients

4 egg whites
8oz caster sugar
1 tablespoon water
1 teaspoon vinegar
½ pint double cream
Kiwi fruit or soft fruit in season

Method

Whip eggs and sugar until firmish. Add water. Whip up, then add vinegar and whip again, the longer the better. Shape into a flan-type base. Put in warm oven at 150°C/300°F (gas mark 2). Leave for 10 minutes, turn gas off and leave pavlova in the oven until cooked. Fill with cream and crown with fruit.

LILIAN COMGARD
Dartford

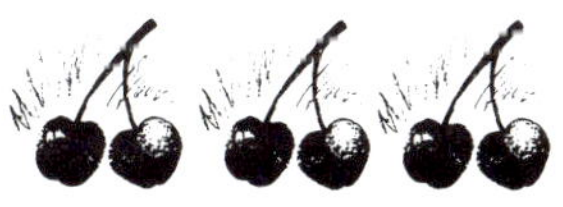

Blackcurrant & Almond Paste Tart

Ingredients

1 egg
6oz caster sugar
1 lemon
8oz ground almonds
6oz icing sugar
Few drops vanilla essence
1lb blackcurrants
Arrowroot and sugar, cooked together

Method

To make almond paste:
Sieve the caster sugar with an equal quantity of icing sugar and mix in a basin with ground almonds and a dessert spoonful of lemon juice. Flavour with a few drops of vanilla essence. Knead the mixture well with the hand until it is smooth, adding beaten egg to moisten as you want it. You can then roll out and fit the flan dish.

Make a deep flan case with almond paste and fill this with blackcurrants which have been stewed in sugar and water. Bind the syrup with a little arrowroot. Eat this flan cold with shortbread fingers or sponge fingers.

PEGGY COLE
Star of Ronald Blyth's film "Akerfield"
Columnist

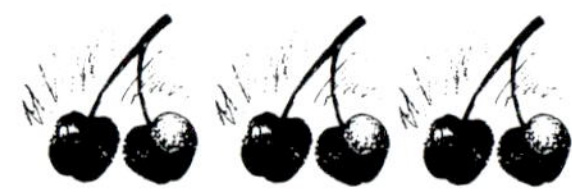

Pineapple Fritters

Ingredients

3oz suet
6oz self-raising flour
1oz caster sugar
1 teaspoon cinnamon
4 pineapple rings
4 cherries
A little milk
Oil for frying

Method

Combine suet, sugar, flour and cinnamon with enough milk to give a firm dough. Roll out thinly and cut into rounds with a saucer. Place a pineapple slice on each round and a cherry in the centre. Brush edges with milk, seal and deep fry until golden.

CHARLES RODGERS

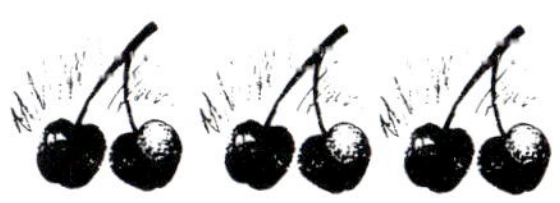

Honey Lemon Cream Pie

Ingredients

2oz butter
4oz digestive biscuits, crushed firmly
1oz soft brown sugar
1 small can evaporated milk
Finely grated rind and juice of 1 lemon
1 tablespoon clear honey
2 tablespoons water
½oz gelatine

Method

Gently melt butter in saucepan, remove from heat and stir in biscuit crumbs and brown sugar. Press around base of a 7″ loose buttered cake tin. Place in fridge to cool for 30 minutes. Pour evaporated milk into large bowl and whisk until very thick and creamy. Add rind and juice of lemon, and honey. Place water in small bowl and sprinkle on gelatine, stir once and leave until spongy, then place bowl in pan of hot water and stir until dissolved. Strain onto honey and lemon mixture. Then pour onto biscuit dish, smoothing surface with a knife. Decorate if desired with a little grated chocolate. Cool in fridge.

This can be open freezed. When frozen, remove pie from tin, wrap in foil, seal and return to freezer. To thaw, unwrap, thaw for about 2 hours at room temperature.

PEGGY ELKINS
Havant, Hampshire

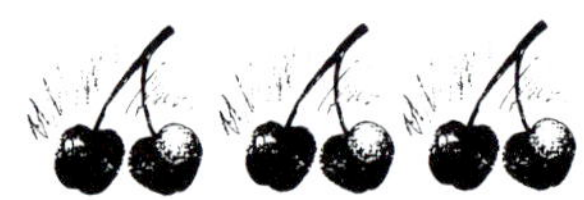

Eve's Pudding

Ingredients & Method

If you wish a good pudding, pray mind what you take,
Two pennyworth of eggs when they're twelve for a groat,
Take of the same fruit which Eve once did cozen,
Well pound and well chopped at least half a dozen,
Six ounces of bread (let your maid eat the crust),
The crumb must be grated as fine as fine dust,
Six ounces of currants, and pray wash them clean,
Lest they grate in your mouth, you know what I mean,
Six ounces of sugar will not make it too sweet,
Some salt and some nutmeg to make it complete,
To this you may add if you are willing and handy,
Some good lemon peel and a large glass of brandy,
Three hours let it boil without hurry or fluster,
And then serve it hot with some good melted butter.

WILTSHIRE F.W.I.

Submitted by
MARLBOROUGH & DISTRICT CARERS GROUP

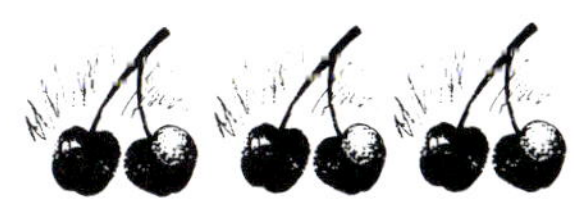

Raspberry Cream Cheese Cake-Tart

Ingredients

1 packet Boudoir biscuits
3fl oz sweet brown sherry
8oz creamed cottage cheese
2 tablespoons caster sugar
6fl oz natural yoghurt
1 packet vanilla instant whip
1oz cornflour
1 can raspberries, drained
8oz cream

Method

Dip biscuits in sherry and place in a layer in dish. Beat cheese, yoghurt, cream, instant whip and sugar. Spread mixture over biscuits. Mix cornflour with raspberry syrup. Pour raspberries and cornflour mixture into saucepan and put on low heat until thick. Cool. Pour over top of pudding and refrigerate until set. Serve with cream.

Comments

I used medium sherry as I did not have sweet sherry. Other toppings – black cherries, strawberries, etc.

CAROLE CLIFFORD

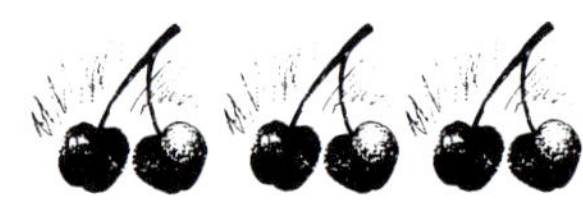

Chocolate Ice Cream

Ingredients

8oz plain chocolate
1 tin condensed milk
8 tablespoons water
1 teaspoon vanilla essence
1 pint double cream

Method

Break chocolate into pieces and place in a basin with the condensed milk. Place over pan of simmering water. When mixture is melted (about 10 minutes) remove from heat. Gradually stir in water and vanilla essence. The mixture becomes thin at this stage. Leave to chill. When cold stir in lightly whipped cream. Blend in thoroughly. Pour into 2 litre polythene container. Freeze until partly frozen. Turn into chilled basin, whisk until creamy and smooth. Return to container and continue to freeze.

THE RT. HON. DAVID MELLOR, MP & HIS SON ANTHONY

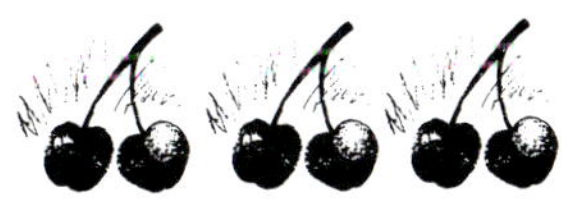

Coffee Mousse

Ingredients

14oz tin evaporated milk
3 tablespoons chocolate powder
¾ breakfast cup strong coffee
2 heaped tablespoons sugar
1 full dessertspoon gelatine

Method

Put half the coffee into a saucepan with gelatine and heat whilst stirring. Mix the chocolate powder and sugar to a stiff paste with the remainder of the coffee. Add the hot coffee and gelatine (*not* boiling). Stir well. Return to the pan and beat again to ensure that everything is dissolved. Do not boil. Allow to cool. Beat evaporated milk until very frothy and thick. Add cold mixture and stir. Pour into a dish to set.

MARTIN MUNCASTER
Writer and Broadcaster

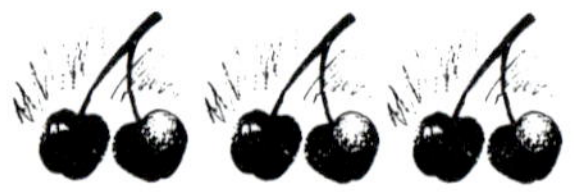

Sussex Pond Pudding

Ingredients

Self-raising flour
Breadcrumbs
Suet
Currants
Butter, unsalted
Demerara sugar
Lemon

Method

Make up enough suet crust to line and cover your chosen pudding basin. Use a mixture of self-raising flour and breadcrumbs (for lightness), half the quantity of grated suet, a handful of currants and enough cold water to bind. Butter the basin. Line with the suet crust reserving enough for the lid. Fill the centre with unsalted butter and demerara sugar, Half a lemon, peel and all, may be added for variety. Top and seal with the remaining suet crust. Cover tightly with greaseproof paper and foil. Steam for at least 2 hours, the longer the better.

To serve, turn the pudding out on to a dish deep enough to contain the buttery sauce which will flow out – hence, *Pond* Pudding.

Comments

Very fattening, very delicious.

JEAN METCALFE

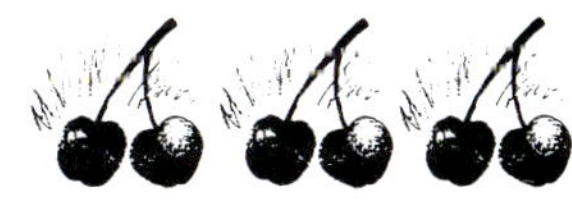

Cazzie's Pud

Ingredients

For cake:

2 cups flour
1 teaspoon baking powder
1½ cups sugar
2 teaspoons bicarbonate of soda
2 eggs
½ teaspoon salt
1 large tin chopped pears
(or fruit cocktail)

For sauce:

1 cup sugar
½ cup dessicated coconut
1 teaspoon vanilla essence
½ cup evaporated milk
4 tablespoons butter

Method

Mix cake ingredients together (add all the juice) and bake at 180°C/350°F (gas mark 4) for 1 hour. Boil the sauce ingredients together and pour over the cake when done.

CAROLE BARROW
Durban, South Africa

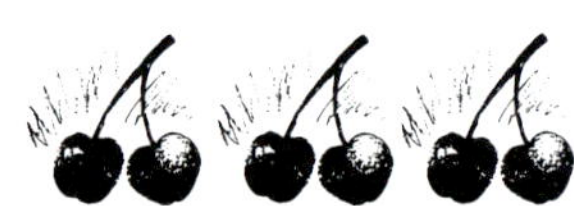

Baked Stuffed Apples

Ingredients

Large eating apples
Raisins (or chopped dates)
1 teaspoon honey

Method

Wash and core one large eating apple for each person. Fill the centre of each apple with raisins or chopped dates. Place a small teaspoonful of honey over the filling. Place in a baking dish and bake in a moderate oven, 180°C/350°F (gas mark 4) until the apples are tender – approximately 35-45 minutes.

To prevent the apples 'exploding', pierce the skin all over with a knife or cook very slowly on a low heat.

Comments

A particular favourite of mine.

ROWAN ATKINSON
Entertainer

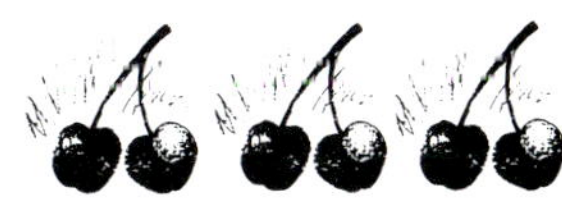

Jellied Kumquats

Ingredients

15oz golden granulated sugar
2lb kumquats
2 tablespoons orange flowerwater
2 packets orange jelly

Method

Bring ¾ pint of water and sugar to boil. Add fruit and simmer until tender – about 30 minutes. Add orange flowerwater and leave to cool. Strain and reserve syrup. Make up jelly incorporating ¾ pint boiled syrup. Pour ½″ of this into mould; set. Put in kumquats with any syrup which sticks to them and cover with remaining jelly. Leave to set. Invert the mould onto a flat plate. Serve with the syrup.

ANNETTE KING
Epping Forest Branch

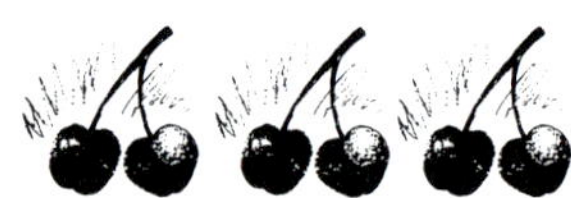

Homemade Marmalade Tart

Ingredients

For pastry:

9oz flour
6oz butter
3oz sugar
1 egg

For filling:

Cream
Homemade marmalade

Method

Make the pastry in the usual way and bake blind. Let it cool. Spread the pastry case with cream that has been stiffened by whipping. Spread the marmalade over the cream in a layer about ½″ deep. Brands such as Golden Shred will not do! Use homemade marmalade, or one of the combined fruit marmalades such as 3-Fruit.

Comments

In my childhood I used to spend odd weekends at the home of my grandparents Augustus and Dorelia John. They lived in a large rambling house at the edge of the New Forest. The kitchen was warmed by an Aga, and there always seemed to be wonderful cooking smells lingering in the passage connecting the kitchen with the dining room. I remember being given marmalade tart for pudding one day. It was, and still is, one of the most delicious things I've ever tasted. I was too young to want the recipe, but here is a version kindly supplied by a family friend, Helen MacDonald-Hall, who lives near Braintree in Essex. Wonderful smells always seem to be wafting out of her kitchen; she too cooks on an Aga.

REBECCA JOHN
London, WC2

Baked Pears with Orange

Ingredients

4 pears
1 large sweet orange
4 tablespoons natural yoghurt or low-fat creme fraîche

Method

Cut pears lengthways and carefully remove core section. Place in oven-proof shallow dish cut side up. Grate orange rind over the pears and squeeze juice over fruit. Bake at 200°C/400°F (gas mark 6), uncovered, for 30 minutes. Serve with yoghurt or low-fat crème fraîche.

PETERBOROUGH BRANCH

Pineapple Delight

Ingredients

1 tin crushed pineapple
1 packet marshmallows
5oz carton of whipping cream

Method

Cut marshmallows into 3 and place in bottom of dish. Pour over marshmallows contents of tin of pineapple. Leave in fridge for 24 hours. Stir mixture. Whip cream and stir into mixture.

VINCENT BILLINGTON
Concert Pianist

Chocolate-Finger Sandwich

Ingredients

2 thick slices of freshly baked white bread
Fresh butter (salted or un-salted)
Chocolate-finger biscuits

Method

Take the slices of bread (of course you can use wholemeal but it's not as much fun or as 'wicked') and spread both generously with butter (of course you can use various spreads low in saturates and cholesterol, high in polyunsaturates, but it's not as much fun etc). Lay several of the chocolate-fingers on one slice, butter-side up. . . place the second slice over the biscuits, butter-side down. . . and you have a delicious, appetising, *wicked* snack!!

Comments

Enjoy!

CHRISTOPHER TIMOTHY
Actor

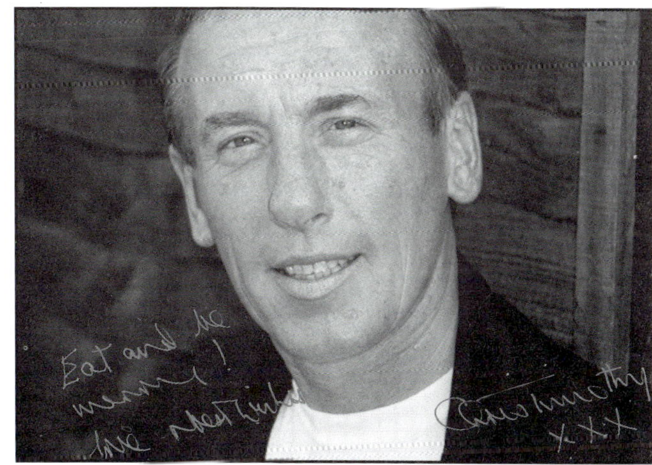

Peach Delight

Ingredients

1 tin sliced peaches (in fruit juice)
Digestive biscuits
Whipping cream

Method

Drain juice from tin of peach slices. Whip cream until stiff. Place two wedges of peach slices on a digestive biscuit forming circle round the biscuit and leaving gap in the middle. Put one teaspoon of cream in centre of peach slices.

SIR CYRIL SMITH, MBE, MP

A Quick Pud

Method

Remove the paper from a Jamaican Cake, place in a covered dish and heat in oven. Make a cornflour sauce adding a teaspoon of ground ginger, and pour over cake. Sprinkle small pieces of crystalised ginger on top.

MARJORIE ROGERS
Stroud

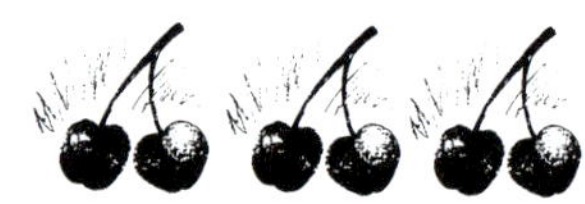

Apple Mousse

Ingredients

1 lime jelly
¼ pint boiling water (approx)
¾ pint stewed apples (approx), sweetened to taste

Method

Melt jelly in about ¼ pint boiling water. When cold add cold stewed apple to bring quantity up to 1 pint. Place in liquidiser or food processor and whizz until blended and smooth. Pour into serving dish and leave to set. Serve with ice cream.

BARBARA KENDALL
Carer, Southsea

Ice Cream & Nuts

Method & Comments

As one who is very busy but equally likes to entertain, I often find myself without a sweet. I have learnt, however, from Italy that a most enjoyable sweet is a good ice cream with honey poured over it and grated nuts. There is therefore no cooking and it can be served in a moment!

THE BARONNESS FAITHFUL, OBE

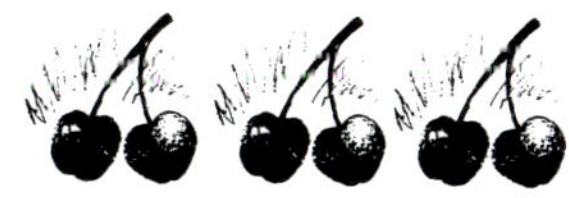

Mum's Egg & Rice Custard

Ingredients

1 pint milk
3 dessertspoons sugar
5 dessertspoons rice
Vanilla essence (to taste)
1 egg

Method

Bring milk and sugar to boil. Shake in rice, boil for 20 minutes, then break in egg and stir vigorously.

Microwave suggestion: Stand container with milk and sugar in a larger bowl to catch the first boil-over, then tip the boil-over back into the container and add rice. Bring to the boil again and immediately switch to defrost for 20 minutes.

ADARDS
Australia

Baked Bananas

Method

Allow two bananas per person. Divide each banana into four by cutting lengthways. Arrange in a shallow oven dish. Cover with orange juice and sprinkle with coconut. Add two knobs of butter. Bake in a medium oven for about 30 minutes.

JO HAWKEY
London, W2

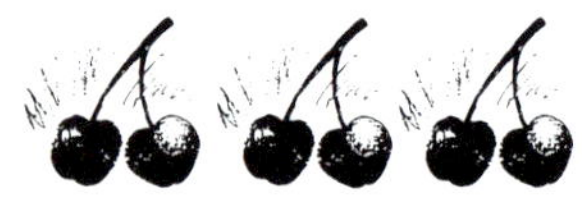

Cakes, Breads & Biscuits

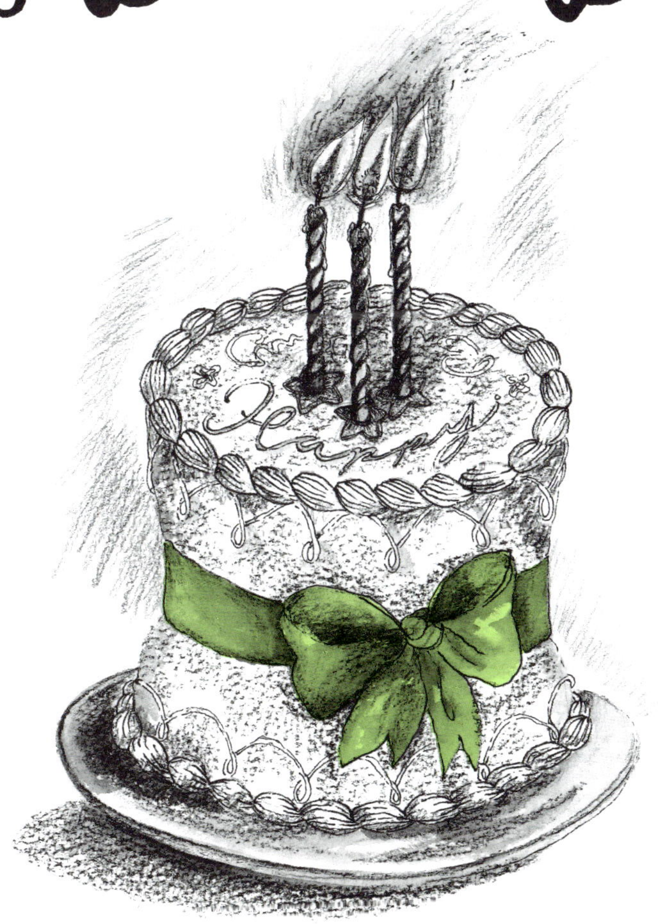

Recipe for Preserving Children

Ingredients

1 grass grown field
A dozen children (or more)
Several dogs (+ puppies if available)
1 brook
Pebbles

Method

Into field, pour children and dogs, allowing to mix well. Pour brook over pebbles till slightly frothy. When children are nicely brown, cool in warm bath. When dry, serve with milk and freshly baked gingerbread.

CHRISTINE WHILD

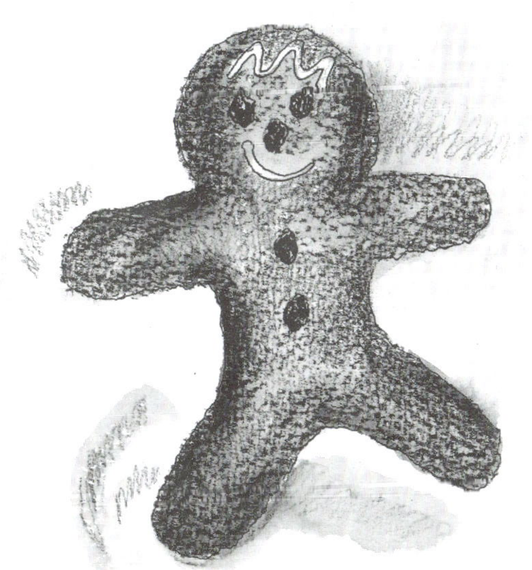

Gingerbread

Ingredients

4oz margarine
6oz black treacle
2oz golden syrup
¼ pint milk
2 eggs
8oz plain flour
2oz sugar
1 rounded teaspoon mixed spice
1 level teaspoon bicarbonate of soda
2 level teaspoons ground ginger

Method

Using a large saucepan warm together margarine, treacle and syrup. Add the milk and allow the mixture to cool.

Beat eggs and add to the cooled mixture. Sieve the dry ingredients together in a bowl, add the cooled mixture and blend together. Turn into a greased and lined 7″ square cake tin.

Bake on the middle shelf of the oven at 160°C/310°F (gas mark 3½) for 1¼-1½ hours.

PETERBOROUGH BRANCH
From their Cookery Book

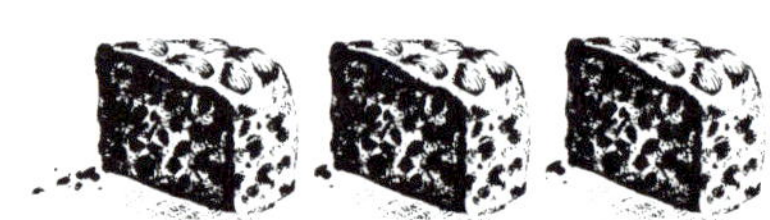

Orange Layer Cake

Ingredients

6oz butter or margarine
6oz caster sugar
4oz cornflour
4oz self-raising flour
3 eggs
6 dessertspoons fresh orange juice

For butter icing (filling):
4oz butter
6oz icing sugar
3 dessert spoons fresh orange juice

For orange icing:
6oz icing sugar
Fresh orange juice to mix

Method

Beat butter and caster sugar together. Add a third of the flour and cornflour mixture, then one egg, then 2 spoonfuls of orange juice, in that order. Repeat twice more. Divide the mixture equally into three greased sandwich tins. Place into pre-heated oven 180°C/350°F (gas mark 4) – one tin on top shelf and two on the shelf below. Cook for about 20 minutes or until golden brown. Leave to cool while you prepare filling and the icing.

Sandwich the three layers together with the filling and top with the icing.

BERYL KINGSTON
Author of "Tuppeny Times", "Fourpenny Flyer" and "Sixpenny Stalls"

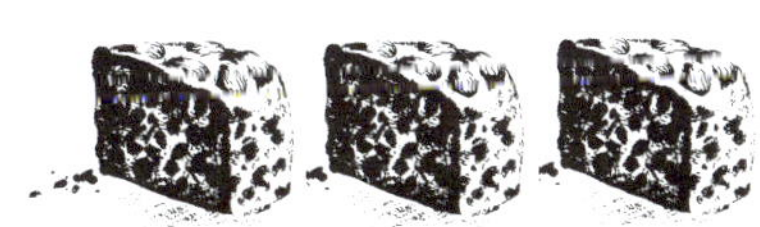

Ginger Biscuit Cake

Ingredients

1 packet ginger nuts
3fl oz sherry (small glass)
1 small carton double cream
1 egg white
1 teaspoon caster sugar
Walnuts and cherries to decorate

Method

Whisk the double cream, egg white and sugar until it is a thick cream and will stand in peaks. Put the sherry into a saucer and dunk the ginger biscuits one at a time into it and sandwich them with cream. Build these up into a small pile. Place this sideways and add to it until you have the length required and then cover all over with cream.

Decorate with cherries and walnuts. You can eat it immediately, but it tastes better if it has been in the fridge for a few hours.

JILL BRANDON

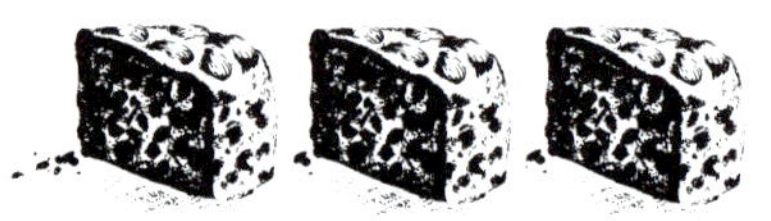

Yorkshire Potato Cakes

Ingredients

1lb potatoes, preferably red-skinned
4oz plain flour
½ teaspoon baking powder
Pinch of salt
2oz butter
¼ pint milk
Butter for serving

Method

Cook and mash potatoes. Sieve flour, baking powder and salt. Rub together the sieved flour and 2oz butter. Add to potatoes and mix into a smooth dough with milk. Roll out the mixture on a floured board to ½″ thickness. Cut into round or square pieces of 4″ in diameter. Bake in a hot oven on a greased tray for 15-20 minutes. Slit open, butter and serve while hot.

Comments

A favourite recipe of mine. The potato cakes can be cooked on a greased griddle or in a frying pan, turning once.

MARIE BELFITT
Local Historian, Scarborough

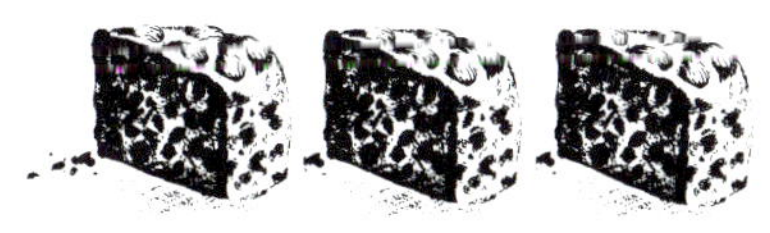

Pineapple Fruit Cake

Ingredients

5oz soft margarine or butter
5oz soft dark brown sugar
2 large beaten eggs
4oz self-raising flour
4oz wholemeal flour
Rind of 1 orange
8oz tin crushed pineapple, drained
10oz raisins
4oz sultanas
2oz cherries, halved
1 dessertspoon golden syrup

Method

Cream fat, sugar, golden syrup and orange rind until light and fluffy. Add beaten eggs and, alternately, flours and dried fruit. Add pineapple, drained. Put in lined 8″ tin. Bake at 170°C/325°F (gas mark 3) for 1¾ hours. Look after 1½ hours and cover if necessary.

A. E. PORT
Twickenham

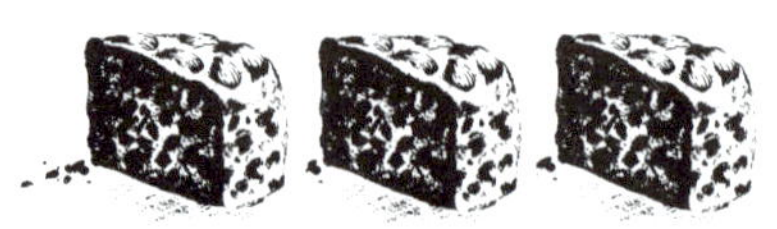

Quark Cake

Ingredients

For base:
6oz crushed digestive biscuits
3oz butter

For topping:
1lb Quark or fromage frais
3oz caster sugar
4 eggs
Grated rind of 2 untreated lemons
1 tablespoon cornflour
2 tablespoons fresh lemon juice

Method

First preheat the oven to 180°C/350°F (gas mark 4). Next lightly grease a loose-bottomed cake tin. Melt the butter gently and add to the crushed biscuits. (I find the easiest way to crush them is inside a polythene bag with a rolling pin.) Press the mixture down firmly into the cake tin to form a smooth base. Beat the Quark and the sugar, stirring continually until the consistency is smooth. Do not use an electric beater, as this makes the Quark too runny. Beat the eggs and stir into the cheese mixture, and then add the lemon rind. Finally, blend the cornflour with the lemon juice and add this to the mixture. Spoon the mixture into the cake tin, and place in the centre of the oven for about 20 minutes. Remove the cheesecake from the oven and chill for several hours. Before serving, decorate with lemon twists.

Comments

Quark is high in protein, and is available in Germany with varying fat contents. "Magerquark" which contains about 3% is ideal for slimmers, while at the other end of the scale is "Sahnequark", with 40% fat content which is rich and creamy

continued

Quark Cake
(cont.)

Comments
(cont.)

and perfect for the not-so-calorie-conscious or "Schlemmer" as they say in Germany. Many large supermarkets in Britain now carry Quark, or a similar French product, Fromage Frais. Both of these have a creamier consistency than regular curd cheese.

When Germans say: "Das ist alles Quark", it means: "That's a load of nonsense". Do not let this put you off Quark, the food!

K. J. LAND
Poole Branch

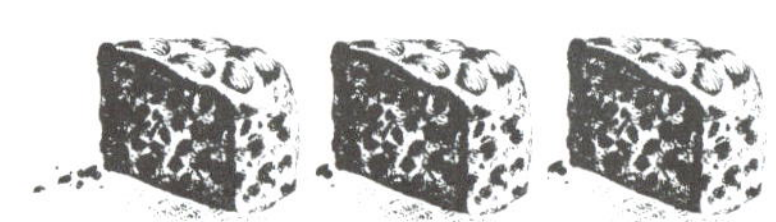

A Special (Birthday) Cake

Ingredients

3 good tablespoons ground coffee
½ pint water
4oz bitter dark chocolate
4oz butter
5oz caster sugar
4 eggs, separated
5oz cornflour
10oz self-raising flour
1 teaspoon salt

Method

Add ground coffee to ½ pint water and reduce by boiling to make ¼ pint of strong coffee. Cool. Grease and line 9″ diameter tin. Heat oven to 180°C/350°F (gas mark 4). Melt chocolate and stir in coffee. Cream butter with caster sugar and add eggs. Combine with chocolate mixture, beating well. Sieve flour and salt, add alternately to mixture with coffee and chocolate. Whisk egg whites till stiff and quickly fold in. Bake for an hour testing to see if sides are shrinking and cake is firm to touch.

Decorate with melted chocolate, or coffee butter icing with walnuts or whipped cream.

MARJORIE ROGERS

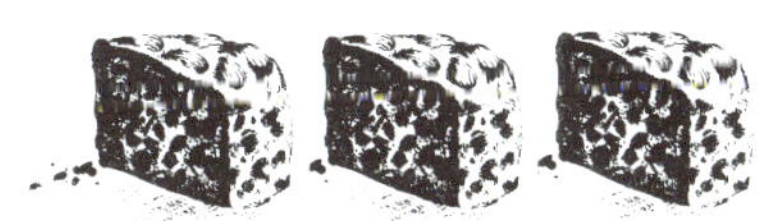

Pineapple & Coconut Brack

Ingredients

15oz can pineapple pieces
5 tablespoons pineapple juice
2oz dessicated coconut
8oz caster sugar
8oz self-raising white flour
2 eggs

Method

Chop pineapple pieces, mix with juice and coconut. Stir in sugar, flour and eggs. Spoon mixture into 2 greased and base-lined 1lb loaf tins. Sprinkle with extra coconut. Cook at 180°C/350°F (gas mark 4) for 40-45 minutes. Test. Turn out and cool. Serve sliced and buttered if liked. Makes twelve 210-calorie slices.

PHYLLIS M. HAYDON
Alzheimer's Widow

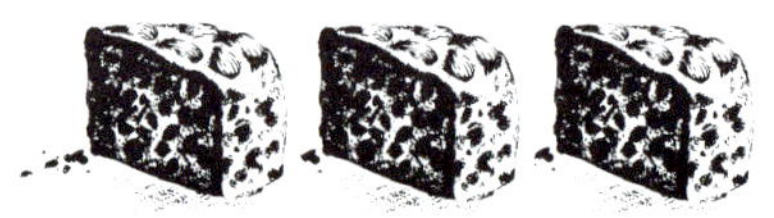

Congress Tarts

Ingredients

Shortcrust pastry

For filling:
3oz caster sugar
3oz margarine
3oz ground rice
Almond essence (1 teaspoon or to taste)
Jam
1 egg, beaten

Method

Make pastry and prepare 12 patty tins. Cream margarine and sugar together and add beaten egg, essence and ground rice. Put a spoonful of jam in each pastry case, then spoon filling on top. (Optional: you can sprinkle a few flaked almonds on top.) Bake for 15-20 minutes at 190°-200°C/375°-400°F (gas mark 6).

ROMFORD & BRENTWOOD SUPPORT GROUP

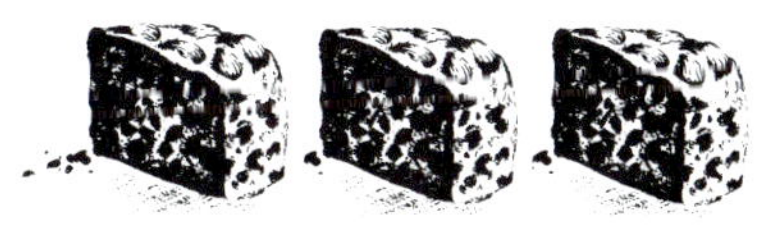

Cheese Twigs

Ingredients

4oz plain flour
Pinch of salt
2oz margarine
3oz coarsely grated cheese
1 crumbled Oxo cube (chicken or beef)
1 egg yolk
2-3 tablespoons water

Method

Rub fat into flour, add salt, stir in cheese. Add Oxo, egg yolk and enough water to mix to firm dough. Turn onto floured board, knead, roll out thinly into large oblong of ¼″ thickness. Cut into ¼″ wide × 3″ long strips. Bake at 200°C/400°F (gas mark 6) for 8-10 minutes. Makes 80.

VICTORIA DAY CENTRE STAFF
Woking Branch

Cooked by their clients under staff supervision.

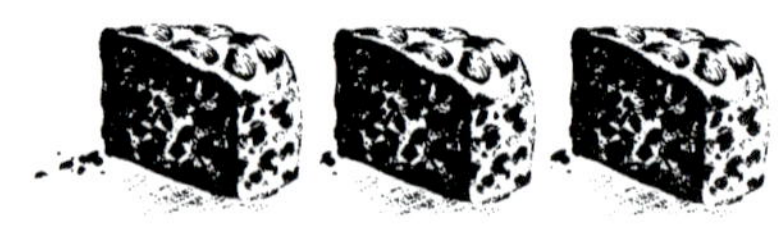

Chocolate Walnut Cakes

Ingredients

4oz dark chocolate
4oz butter
12oz caster sugar
1 teaspoon vanilla essence
2 eggs, lightly beaten
4oz self-raising flour sifted with ½ teaspoon salt
4-6oz walnuts, crushed

Method

Butter and line an 8″ square tin. Soften chocolate in bowl over hot water. Beat in butter away from heat. Beat in sugar and essence. Beat in eggs a little at a time. Quickly stir in flour and salt, and stir in nuts. Spoon and spread evenly in cake tin. Bake at 180°C/350°F (gas mark 4) for 35-40 minutes. Allow to cool slightly and cut into squares. Store in airtight tin. Makes 16. Can be frozen.

B. H. ROSTANCE

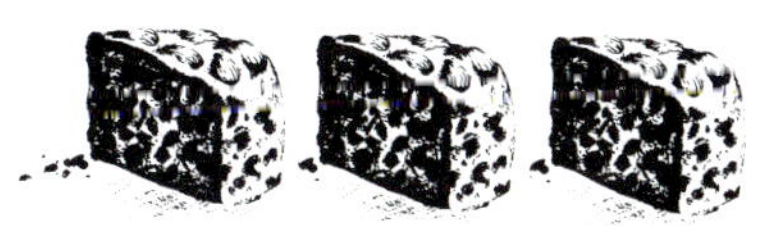

Scottish Shortbread

Ingredients

5oz self-raising flour
2oz caster sugar
1oz rice flour
4oz butter
Pinch of salt

Method

Sieve dry ingredients together. Divide butter into two. Work one half into dry ingredients and allow the other half to melt into 8″ tin as oven is warming up. Use the melted butter to mix in with other ingredients. Knead well until quite smooth.

Press into baking tin working dough neatly into sides and corners. Prick with a fork. Bake in moderate oven at 170°C/325°F (gas mark 3) for 10-15 minutes. Then reduce to 150°C/300°F (gas mark 2) for the rest of the hour. Cut into portions immediately after it is taken out of oven. But leave in tin to cool. Dust with a little fine sugar.

ELSIE C. HARRIS

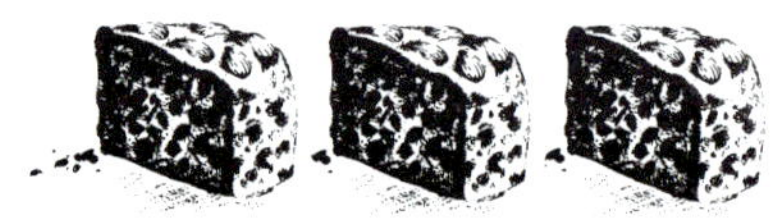

Lardy Cake

Ingredients

8oz flour
¼ teaspoon salt
¼ teaspoon mixed spice
¼oz yeast
1 teaspoon sugar
¼ pint warm milk
2oz lard
2oz sugar
2oz dried fruit

Method

Warm the flour, salt and spice. Cream the yeast with 1 teaspoon sugar. Add the creamed yeast to the flour and mix with enough warm milk to make a soft dough. Beat well. Cover and stand aside in a warm place until twice the size.

Roll out on a well floured board to ¼″ thickness. Spread on half the lard, sugar and fruit. Fold in three, turn the mixture to the left as for flaky pastry and roll out again. Cover with the rest of the lard, sugar and fruit. Again fold in three. Roll out into an oblong 1″ thick.

Place on a deep tin and stand in a warm place until well risen. Score the top with a knife. Brush with sugar and water. Cook in a hot oven for about 30 minutes.

MARLBOROUGH & DISTRICT CARERS GROUP

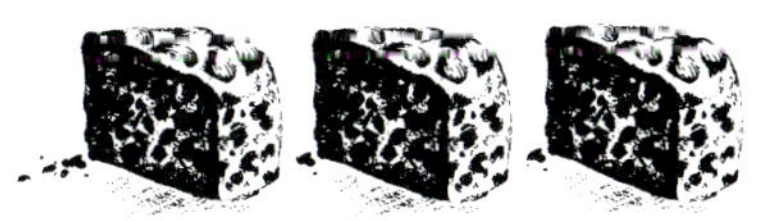

Sherry Biscuits

Ingredients

5oz plain flour
4oz butter or margarine
3oz caster sugar
1 egg
1 tablespoon sherry
Chopped almonds

Method

Sift flour and rub in fat. Add sugar, egg yolk and sherry to make a stiff dough. Roll out to $^1/_8$″ thick. Prick with a fork and cut into fancy shapes with a 2″ cutter. Brush biscuits with lightly beaten egg white and sprinkle with chopped almonds. Bake in oven at 180°C/350°F (gas mark 4) for 15 minutes. Makes about 30 biscuits.

CHARLES RODGERS
Dartford Branch

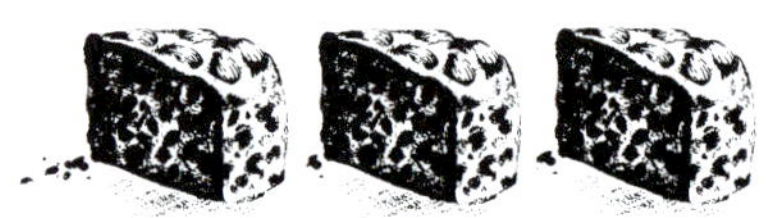

Carrot Cake

Ingredients

4oz grated carrot
5oz soft brown sugar
8oz self-raising flour
2 level teaspoon baking powder
2oz chopped nuts
2 eggs
¼ pint corn oil

For topping:
3oz margarine
3oz Philadelphia cream cheese
6oz icing sugar
¼ teaspoon vanilla essence

Method

Mix all ingredients together with oil and place in a 2lb loaf tin which has been greased and lined with grease-proof paper. Cook at 180°C/350°F (gas mark 4) for 1¼ hours. Mix topping ingredients until creamy. Place on top of cake when cake is fully cooled.

Comments

Always a winner at that special tea party. Keeps well in fridge.

KATHY GRANT
Jersey

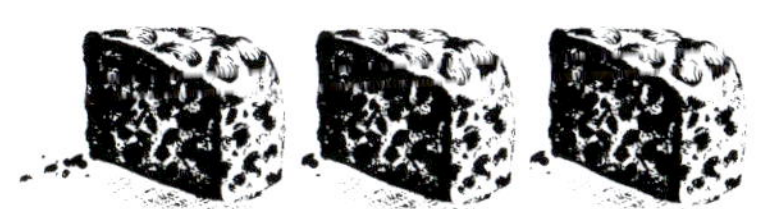

Banana & Walnut Loaf

Ingredients

7oz self-raising flour
1 level teaspoon baking powder
2oz walnuts, finely chopped
1 tablespoon cube sugar, crushed
1oz lard
3oz caster sugar
2 large bananas, mashed
4fl oz milk

Method

Mix together flour and baking powder. Rub lard into flour, add sugar and walnuts. Stir in bananas and milk and mix to a stiff consistency. Turn into a greased 1lb loaf tin. Sprinkle top with crushed cube sugar and bake at 190°C/375°F (gas mark 5) for 1½ hours. Turn out and cool. Slice and serve buttered. Flavour improves with freezing.

Comments

To serve from freezer, thaw wrapped overnight or for 3-4 hours at room temperature.

ROMFORD & BRENTWOOD SUPPORT GROUP

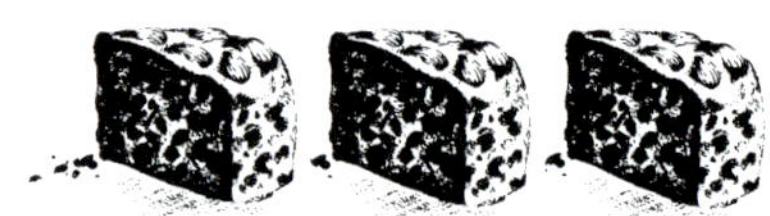

Picnic Slices

Ingredients

8oz block milk chocolate
2oz butter or margarine
4oz caster sugar
4oz dessicated coconut
2oz sultanas
2oz chopped glacé cherries
1 egg, beaten

Method

Break chocolate into pieces and melt in a basin over pan of hot water. Pour into bottom of a greased Swiss roll tin. Allow to set. Cream fat and sugar, add egg, fruit and coconut. Mix well and spread over the set chocolate.

Bake near bottom of a slow oven till golden brown – if oven is too hot the top will burn. After cooling slightly mark into slices. Leave till cold and then cut out of tin.

DORA ALLENGAME
Bognor Regis & District Carers Group

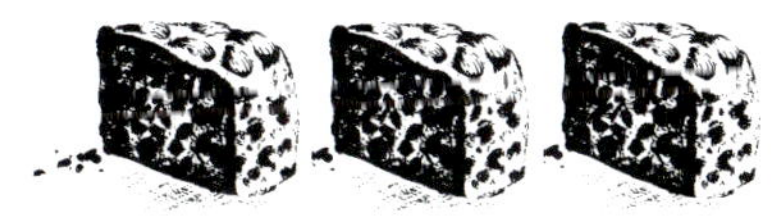

Semolina Crisps

Ingredients

4oz flour
2oz semolina
2oz caster sugar
4oz margarine
1 tablespoon golden syrup
1 small teaspoon bicarbonate of soda
1 teaspoon ground ginger
Pinch of salt

Method

Cream fat and sugar together in warm basin with syrup. Mix all dry ingredients together and add to creamed fat mixture. This forms a stiff paste. Flour hands and roll into balls about the size of walnuts. Place on a greased tray well apart and bake in a moderate oven at 180°C/350°F (gas mark 4) for about 10 minutes until golden brown.

JOAN ROBERTS
Chichester Branch

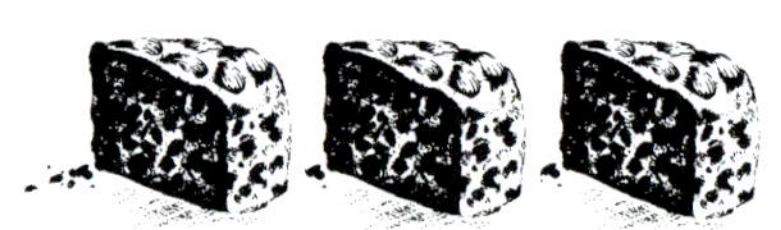

Cumberland Lemon Pastry Cake

Ingredients

12oz shortcrust pastry (for two cakes)

For filling:

½lb caster sugar
Rind and juice of 1 lemon
2 eggs, beaten
2oz butter or margarine

Method

Line two plate cake tins with half of the shortcrust pastry. Mix all filling ingredients together, and divide the mixture between the two cakes. Dot small piece of margarine onto each cake, moisten edges, and prick. Roll out the second half of the pastry and cover the cakes. Seal edges. Bake at 200°C/400°F (gas mark 6) for 20-30 minutes.

PENRITH SUPPORT GROUP

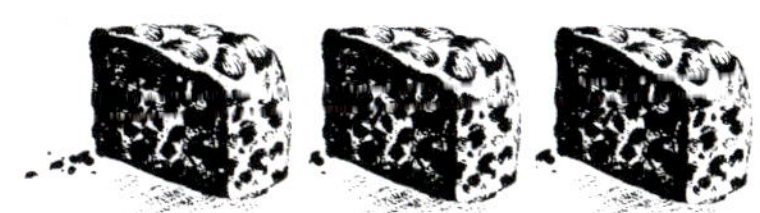

Welsh Cakes

Ingredients

8oz self-raising flour
4oz block margarine
3oz dried fruit
3oz sugar
1 egg
Pinch of mixed spice

Method

Rub margarine into flour, add sugar, fruit and spice. Beat egg, pour into mixture and mix to firm dough. Roll out to ½″ thick, cut into rounds. Cook on griddle for about 3 minutes each side, turning only once. Sprinkle with caster sugar.

NEATH & PORT TALBOT BRANCH

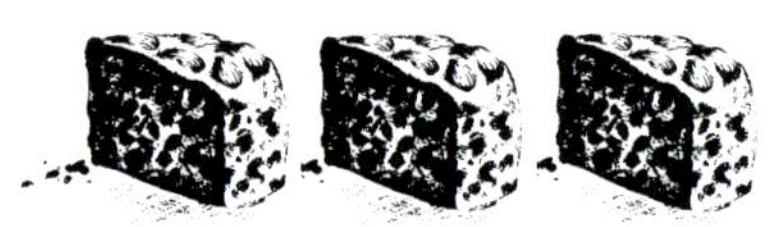

Coconut & Chocolate Fingers

Ingredients

2oz margarine
2oz walnuts, chopped
4oz dessicated coconut
4oz sugar
4oz glacé cherries
1 egg
8oz cooking chocolate, milk or plain

Method

Line Swiss roll tin with greaseproof paper. Melt chocolate. Spread over paper in tin and leave to set.

Cream margarine and sugar, add beaten egg and other ingredients. Spread over chocolate and bake in moderate oven 180°C/350°F (gas mark 4) for 20 minutes. Leave to cool – cut into fingers before chocolate sets.

SIR JAMES ANDERTON
Chief Constable, Greater Manchester

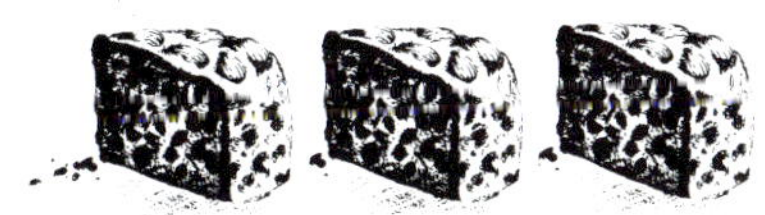

Granma's Cookies
(COLUMBUS OHIO)

Ingredients

¾ cup sugar
1 cup margarine
2 cups flour
2 cups rolled oats
1 cup raisins
2 eggs
5 tablespoons raisin juice
1 teaspoon bicarbonate of soda
2 teaspoons cinnamon
1 teaspoon vanilla
1 packet chocoloate chips

Method

Cook raisins in 1 cup of water and drain. Reserve the water.

Mix together all ingredients except for chocolate chips. Bind with raisin juice until the mixture is soft. Mix in the chocolate chips.

Drop heaped teasponsfuls on to greased baking sheet. Cook in moderate oven 200°C/400°F (gas mark 6) for 15-20 minutes.

ROSEMARY REODER

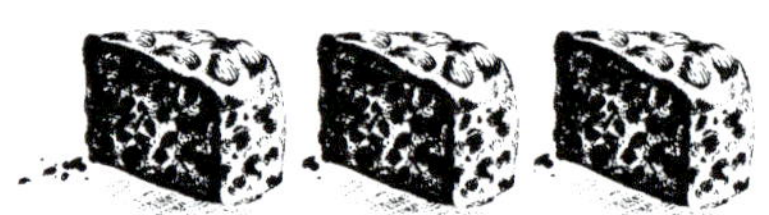

Cumbrian Treacle Bread

Ingredients

2lb wholemeal flour
1oz dried yeast or 2oz fresh yeast
¼ pint warm water
2 tablespoons treacle
½oz salt
3oz cracked wheat or bran

Method

Stir the treacle into the ¼ pint of warm water, sprinkle the yeast on top, and put in a warm place until a nice froth has formed (7 to 10 minutes). Add the yeast mixture to the dry ingredients and mix well. Divide between 4 1lb loaf tins, greased. Press down with your hand – the mixture will be sticky so dampen your hand – and leave to rise in a warm place for about 40 minutes. Bake at 200°C/400°F (gas mark 6) for 30 minutes. Bake for a further 5 minutes for a nice crisp loaf.

Comments

So easy to make. Must be – I now make it myself every Sunday morning, just to hear the rest of the family going yum yum!

HUNTER DAVIES

Submitted by
Dawn Marriott

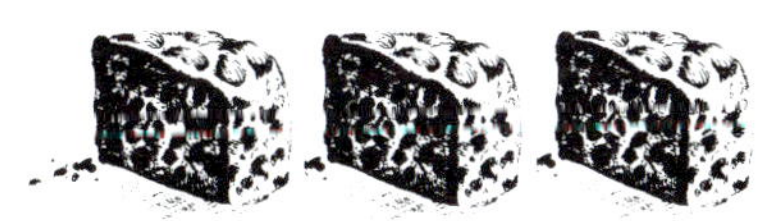

The Queen Mother's Date & Walnut Cake

Ingredients

8oz sugar
3oz margarine
1 egg, beaten
1 teaspoon vanilla essence
10oz self-raising flour
1 teaspoon bicarbonate of soda
1 teaspoon salt
8oz dates
2oz walnuts, chopped

Method

Pour ½ pint of boiling water over 8oz chopped dates. Add 1 teaspoon bicarbonate of soda and leave to stand while mixing the other ingredients. Add this mixture to date mixture and cook for approx 35 minutes in a moderate oven, in a tin measuring 12″ × 9″.

Comments

I bought this recipe in Scotland many years ago on the understanding that it was allowed only to be sold for charity – I have seen it in one other Charity Cookery Book since.

WENDY DITCHAM
South West Branch Regional Office, Bath

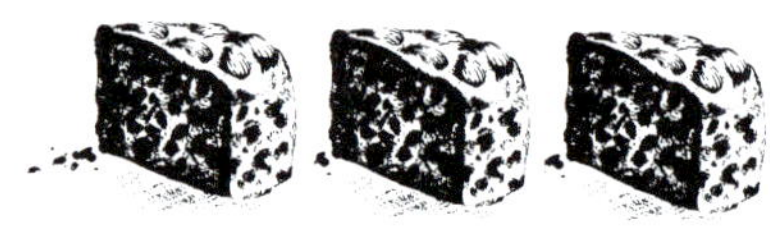

Foursies

Ingredients

3oz butter
1oz sugar
8oz plain flour
¼ teaspoon bicarbonate of soda
¼ teaspoon cream tartar
1 large egg
Water

Method

Cream butter and sugar together. Sift flour, bicarbonate of soda and cream of tartar. Add egg to creamed mixture alternately with the flour. Mix with a little water if needed to form a stiffish dough. Roll out onto a floured board until ¼″ to ½″ thick. Using a 2″ cutter stamp out rounds. Bake for about 10 minutes at 180°C/350°F (gas mark 4). Slice in half horizontally and bake cut side up for a further 10 minutes. Cool on wire tray, serve with butter or cream cheese. Makes about 30.

Comments

Traditional Suffolk recipe which is eaten in the fields by farmworkers when they take a break from ploughing.

PAUL HEINEY
BBC Television

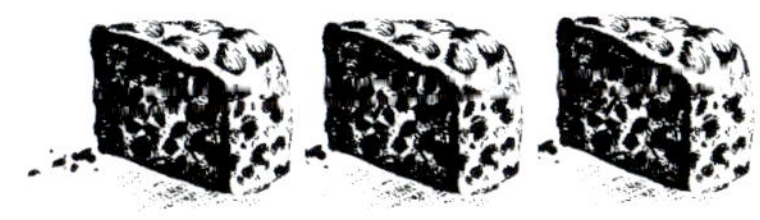

Wholefood Mincemeat Slices

Ingredients

5oz vegetable margarine
3oz soft brown sugar
8oz wholewheat flour
4oz porridge oats
8oz mincemeat

Method

You'll need a shallow baking tin 11″ × 7″, well buttered.

Start by melting the margarine gently in a large saucepan, together with the brown sugar. While that's happening, mix the flour and porridge oats together in a mixing bowl. When the margarine and sugar mixture has become liquid and there are no lumps or fat or sugar lurking (give it a stir with a wooden spoon to get rid of them), remove the pan from the heat and begin adding the flour and oats to the pan, stirring well with each addition.

When it's all thoroughly blended, spoon half the mixture into the prepared tin. Now, using the flat of your hand, press the mixture down firmly all over, making sure it gets into all the corners. The firmer you press, the less crumbly the slices will be when they're cooked.

Next, using a tablespoon, spread the mincemeat evenly all over, pressing it out with the back of the spoon. Then spread the remaining oat mixture over the top, again pressing it down firmly and evenly all over.

Now bake the mixture in the centre of the oven for about 20 minutes or until the top is tinged brown. Then remove it from the oven and use a sharp knife to cut

continued

Wholefood Mincemeat Slices (cont.)

Method (cont.)

it into 12 squares, but leave them in the tin until they are quite cold. Then you can remove them more easily.

When they've cooled, lift them out with a palette knife and store in an airtight tin – that's if they are not all eaten straight away!

DELIA SMITH
From her recently published "Christmas Book"

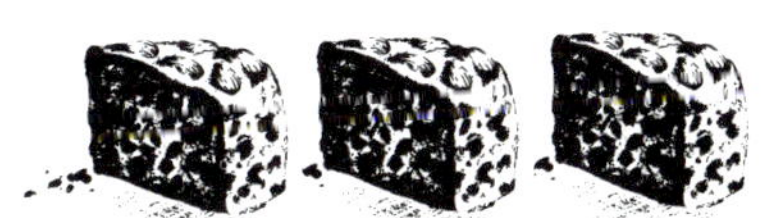

Lemon Cake

Ingredients

4oz soft margarine
6oz self-raising flour
1 level teaspoon baking powder
6oz caster sugar
2 eggs
4 tablespoons milk
Rind from 1 lemon

For glaze:
Juice of 1 lemon
4oz granulated sugar

For lemon butter cream filling:
3oz margarine
6oz icing sugar
A few drops of lemon juice

Method

Beat all the ingredients thoroughly and bake in a greased, lined cake tin. Bake at 170°C/325°F (gas mark 3) for about 1 hour.

Squeeze the juice from 1 lemon and mix with 4oz granulated sugar. When the cake is cooked and still hot, pour the sugar and lemon juice over it. When cold, remove cake from tin. Make butter cream.

Slice the cake in half and fill with lemon butter cream.

DR CHRIS STOCKDALE
Family Doctor and Marathon Swimmer

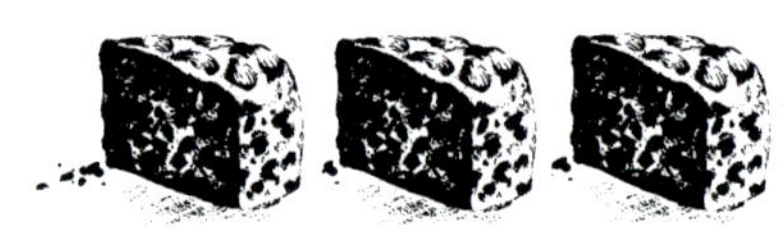

Drop Scones

Ingredients

4oz self-raising flour
½oz margarine
2oz sugar
1 egg
4 tablespoons milk
Pinch of salt
Oil for griddle or frying pan

Method

Sieve flour and salt into bowl. Rub in margarine. Stir in sugar. Beat egg and milk together and add to flour mixture a little at a time, beating with a whisk until smooth.

Heat griddle or frying pan, with a little oil in it. Drop tablespoons of the mixture into the griddle or into the pan and cook for about 3 minutes until tiny bubbles appear and burst. Turn with a palette knife and cook the other side until golden brown.

When cooked pile the scones in a clean tea towel to keep warm and moist. Serve as soon as possible.

VALERIE SINGLETON

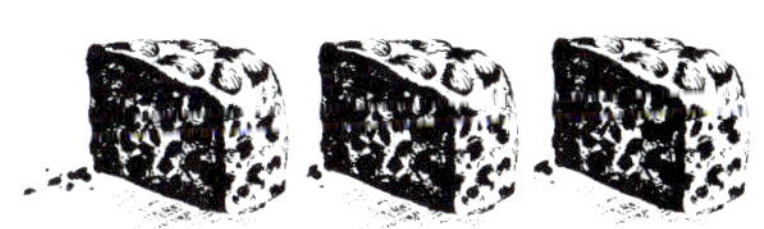

Gooey Chocolate Cake

Ingredients

4oz plain dessert chocolate
4oz softened butter
4oz caster sugar
3 eggs
2oz ground almonds
¼ teaspoon almond essence
2oz plain flour

To serve:
Sifted icing sugar
Whipped cream
Strawberries

Method

Pre-heat oven to 180°C/350°F (gas mark 4). Grease an 8″ springform cake tin and dust with some caster sugar.

Melt chocolate with two tablespoonfuls of water in a bowl over a pan of hot water. Cool.

Cream butter with sugar till pale and fluffy. Beat in egg yolks, one at a time. Fold melted chocolate, almonds and essence into mixture. Whip egg white until stiff. Fold in one rounded tablespoon egg white, then the flour, followed by the remaining egg white until evenly blended.

Spread into prepared tin, smooth the top and bake in the centre of the oven for 35 minutes until the outer edges are firm but the centre is still slightly soft. The secret of the cake is the gooey, slightly underdone centre. Slightly cool the cake in tin then turn out onto a wire rack. Leave until cold. Dust liberally with icing sugar.

Serve each slice with a dollop of whipped cream and add a few strawberries.

SIR STANLEY BAILEY
Chief Constable Northumbria Police, Newcastle

Blackberry Crackle Cake

Ingredients

8oz self-raising flour, sieved with a pinch of salt
2oz margarine
4oz caster sugar
1 teaspoon vanilla essence
1 large egg, beaten
4fl oz cold milk
4oz blackberries
1 level teaspoon ground cinnamon
1 extra tablespoon caster sugar

Method

Cream the margarine, sugar and vanilla essence until they are light and fluffy. Beat in the egg. Gradually add the flour and the milk. Put the mixture in a greased 8″ sandwich tin and cover it with blackberries. Mix the cinnamon with the extra sugar and sprinkle it over the top.

Bake for ¾-1 hour at 190°C/375°F (gas mark 5). Cool in the tin and cut into wedges when cold. Serve with whipped cream.

Serves 8.

MRS YVONNE BALCHIN
From Jimmy Young Show

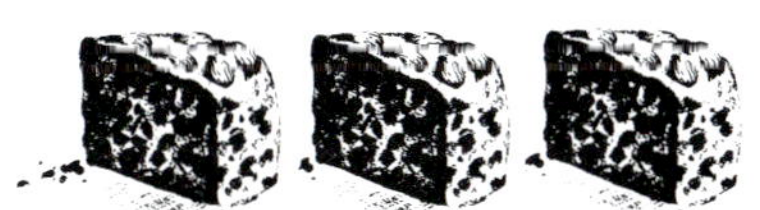

Easy Farmhouse Fruit Cake

Ingredients

6oz demerara sugar
5oz sultanas
4oz currants
5oz seedless raisins
10fl oz water
3oz glacé cherries
4oz butter or margarine

1 egg, beaten
Pinch of salt
10oz sieved self-raising flour
2oz blanched almonds
Optional:
1 teaspoon ginger, ½ teaspoon mixed spice, ½ teaspoon nutmeg

Method

Put fruit, sugar, water, butter and cherries into a saucepan and bring to the boil, then simmer for 20 minutes. Pour mixture into mixing bowl and cool.

Preheat oven to 170°C/325°F (gas mark 3). Grease and line an 8″ round cake tin.

Add egg to cooled mixture and stir well. Finally add flour and spices if using, and mix well. Turn into cake tin, smooth top and arrange almonds on top. Bake 1¼-1½ hours until well risen and golden. Cool before turning out.

MRS B. M. PURDUE

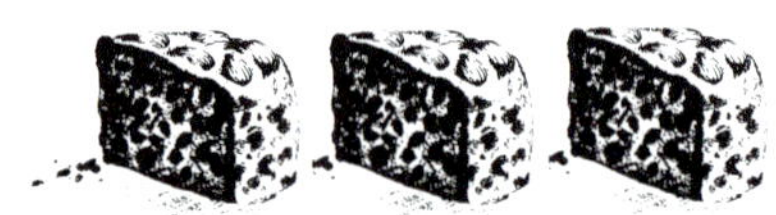

Yorkshire Fruit Loaf

Ingredients

8oz sultanas
4oz mixed peel
¼ teaspoon salt
8oz sugar
¼ pint milk
8oz currants
1lb self-raising flour
8oz margarine
2 eggs
½ teaspoon bicarbonate of soda

Method

Wash fruit and dry. Chop peel. Sieve flour with salt and mix in margarine until it forms fine breadcrumbs. Stir in sugar and fruit. Beat eggs and add bicarbonate of soda in a little milk. Divide mixture into 2 tins. Bake in moderate oven 190°C/ 375°F (gas mark 5) for approx 60 minutes.

MARY CALLAND
Secretary, Ryhl Branch

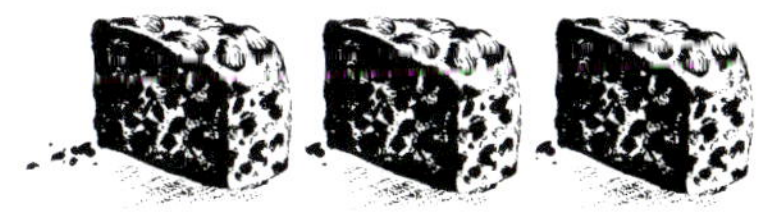

Long-Keeping Fruit Cake

Ingredients

6oz butter
6oz sugar (brown molasses is excellent)
3 eggs beaten
8oz plain flour
½ teaspoon baking powder
1lb mixed dried fruit
2oz glacé cherries
2oz peel, sliced and a little grated lemon or orange peel if liked
4oz ground almonds
Brandy

Method

Cream together butter and sugar. Beat in eggs gradually. Sieve flour with baking powder and fold into mixture. Stir dried fruit, cherries, peel and almonds into mixture.

Put into lined 9″ or 10″ cake tin. Bake at 150°C/300°F (gas mark 2) for 1 hour or at 140°C/275°F (gas mark 1) for 1½ hours. When cooked allow a little brandy to soak in.

MARJORIE ROGERS

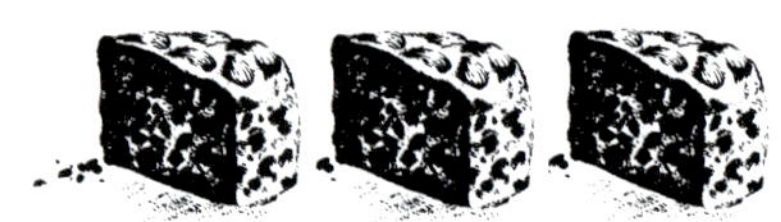

Tea Bread

Ingredients

8oz sultanas, raisins or mixed fruit
8oz finely grated carrots
5fl oz hot black tea
8oz flour
1 medium egg
1 teaspoon mixed spice or cinnamon
½oz granulated or powder sweetener

Method

Soak fruit and carrots overnight in tea. Preheat oven to 170°C/325°F (gas mark 3). Stir flour, egg, spice and sweetener into fruit mixture. Spoon into a greased and lined 2lb loaf tin. Cook for 1½ hours (or until skewer comes out clean) until crusty on top. Cool in tin. Turn out onto wire rack. Mark top evenly into 16 slices.

Comments

Fat and sugar free.

COLCHESTER STANWAY TOWNSWOMEN'S GUILD

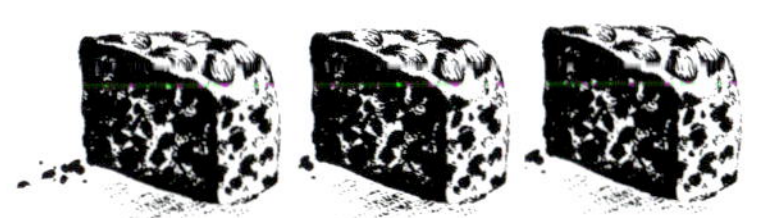

Fruit Cake

Ingredients

1lb plain flour
6oz margarine
7oz caster sugar
6oz sultanas
6oz currants
3oz cherries
2 level teaspoons bicarbonate of soda
½ pint milk
3 tablespoons malt vinegar

Method

Rub margarine into flour, add sugar and fruit. Mix bicarbonate of soda in milk, and add to the mixture. Beat well, stir in vinegar, beat quickly and spoon into 7″ greased cake tin. Bake in moderate oven for 2 hours. After 1 hour cover top with grease-proof paper and check after 1½ hours. Halve quantities for small loaf tin and bake 45 minutes to 1 hour.

Comments

Very nice cut in slices and spread with butter.

MARY HEDDINGTON
Dartford Branch

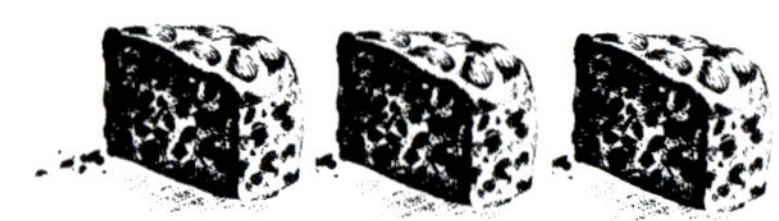

Parkin

Ingredients

¾ tin golden syrup
½ cup milk
4oz margarine
4oz lard
8oz self-raising flour
8oz oatmeal
4oz sugar
1 teaspoon ground ginger

Method

Melt syrup, milk, margarine and lard. Mix the dry ingredients together, then stir in syrup mixture. Beat well. Put in a well greased tin and bake at 190°C/375°F (gas mark 5) for about an hour.

BARNSLEY BRANCH

Date & Walnut Fingers

Ingredients

4oz margarine
7oz self-raising flour
4oz sugar
8oz chopped dates
2oz chopped walnuts
1 egg

Method

Melt the margarine and stir in the other ingredients. Spread mixture in a baking tin and cook in a moderate oven for 20 minutes.

FIONA GOW

Audrey's Gingies

Ingredients

2 level breakfast cups plain flour
1 heaped breakfast cup soft brown sugar
8oz butter
2 teaspoons ginger

Method

Rub the softened butter into the other ingredients as you would for pastry. Put the mixture into a 1″ deep baking tin. Bake for 25 minutes at 170°C/325°F (gas mark 3). Leave to cool for a little time and then cut into squares.

AUDREY LEES
South West London Relatives' Support Group

Home-Made Biscuits

Ingredients

8oz plain flour
8oz self-raising flour
8oz sugar
8oz margarine
Knob of butter
1 tablespoon golden syrup
1oz almonds

Method

Cream margarine, butter, sugar and golden syrup. Mix in flour and knead. Chop or slice almonds and mix in. Roll with hands into a long sausage shape. Cut into rounds. Bake for 20 minutes at 190°C/375°F (gas mark 5).

STEVE WHITE
National Membership Officer

Oat Crunchies

Ingredients

2oz margarine
2oz cooking fat
3oz sugar
4oz self-raising flour
1 teacup porridge oats
1 teaspoon baking powder
1 teaspoon syrup
3 teaspoons boiling water

Method

Put water and syrup in a bowl, work in all the remaining ingredients. Roll into small balls, place on a slightly greased tray and bake for 15-20 minutes at 190°C/375°F (gas mark 5).

JOSIE THORN
Bognor Regis & District Carers Group

Quick & Easy Malt Bread

Ingredients

8oz self-raising flour
3oz brown sugar (preferably demerara)
1 tablespoon black treacle
1 teaspoon baking powder
1 cup water
Handful dried fruit
Pinch of salt

Method

Mix all dry ingredients, including fruit. Add treacle and enough water to make a loose mixture. Put in loaf tin and bake at 180°C/350°F (gas mark 4) for 1 hour.

DAWN MARRIOTT
Camden Support Group

Biscuit Cake

Ingredients

8oz Rich Tea biscuits, crushed
4oz margarine
½oz cocoa powder
2oz sugar
1 tablespoon golden syrup
4oz plain chocolate

Method

Heat the margarine, cocoa powder, sugar and syrup until melted. Add the crushed biscuit and mix. Spread into a shallow tin and press it down well (approx ½″ deep). Melt the chocolate and spread it over the biscuit mixture.

Leave to cool/solidify and cut into 1″ to 2″ squares.

Comments

Taken from the *Winnie the Pooh Cook Book* and known with much love and reverence as 'Pooh Cake'!

JON CLAPHAM
Newcastle Weather Centre

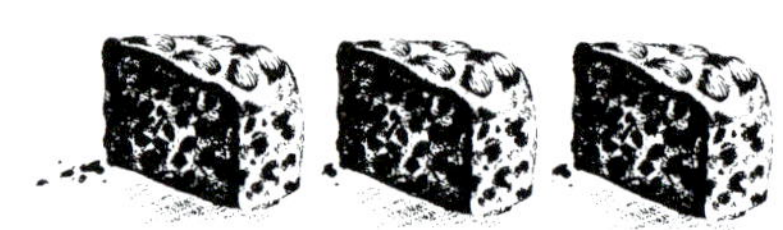

Granny Cowell's Yorkshire Scones

Ingredients

10oz self-raising flour
2oz margarine
2oz sugar
2oz sultanas
2 eggs
A little milk

Method

Rub margarine into flour, add sugar and sultanas. Beat eggs and add to mixture with a little milk (saving a little to brush onto the tops of the scones) to make a soft dough. Roll the mixture into a long sausage and divide into 16. Place each piece on a flat well greased baking tin, brush the tops with the egg and milk, then pop into a hot oven (middle shelf), 210°C/425°F (gas mark 7) for 15-20 minutes, until golden brown.

When the scones are baked, take out of oven and leave to cool. Cover with a clean teacloth.

LEICESTER BRANCH

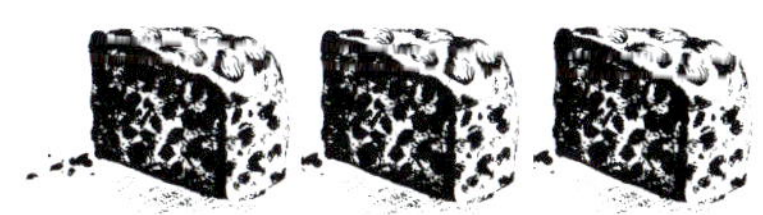

Anzacs

Ingredients

4oz butter or margarine
3 teaspoons golden syrup
¾ teacup sugar
1 teaspoon bicarbonate of soda
2 tablespoons boiling water
¾ teacup flour
1 teacup dessicated coconut
1 teacup walnuts, chopped

Method

Warm fat, syrup and sugar in a fairly large saucepan. Add the soda mixed with the boiling water. Add remaining ingredients and mix all to a moist, but firm, consistency. Heap the mixture in small piles on cold baking trays. Bake in a slow oven at 150°C/300°F (gas mark 2) for 30 minutes, until golden brown.

MEG SKINNER
National Office, Alzheimer's Disease Society, Balham

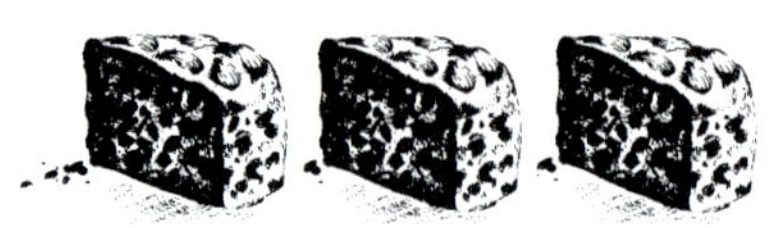

One Stage Marmalade Cake

Ingredients

4oz soft tub margarine
4oz caster sugar
4oz self-raising flour
2 eggs
3 tablespoons chunky marmalade
Water to mix

Method

Place margarine, sugar, eggs, flour, marmalade and water in a bowl and beat well with a wooden spoon for 2-3 minutes until well blended. Turn mixture into an 8″ well greased and base lined double depth sandwich tin and bake at 180°C/ 350°F (gas mark 4) for 35-40 minutes.

Comments

This is a nice cut-and-come-again cake, but can be made more special by the addition of a thin layer of marmalade to the top, and over that a layer of glacé icing.

JOAN M PLATTS
Secretary, Watford & District Branch

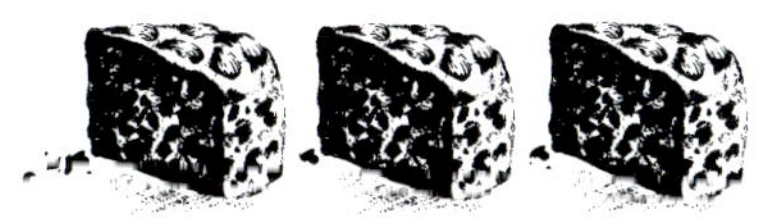

No-Cook Chocolate Cake

Ingredients

8oz digestive biscuits
4oz soft brown sugar
4oz butter
2oz raisins
3 tablespoons cocoa powder
1 egg, beaten
A few drops of vanilla essence

Method

Chop biscuits coarsely. Place sugar and butter in a pan and heat gently until melted, then add the raisins and cocoa. Remove from heat and add the egg and vanilla essence. Pour this mixture onto the biscuits and mix well. Chill in the refrigerator until set.

Comments

For extra special treats, cover with melted cooking or Bourneville chocolate and also add walnuts and cherries to biscuit mix. Another special extra – soak the raisins in rum first.

JOHN TIMPSON
Broadcaster

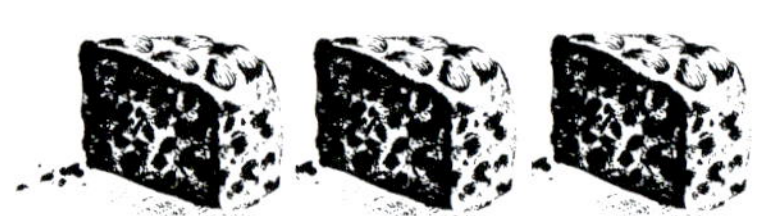

Syrup Oaties

Ingredients

4oz soft vegetable margarine
2 tablespoons golden syrup
8oz oats

Method

Lightly grease 2 baking trays and heat oven to 190°C/375°F (gas mark 5). Melt syrup and margarine over a low heat. Stir together in a bowl with oats. Place large teaspoonfuls of mixture onto trays. Flatten with back of fork and bake for 12 minutes or till golden brown. Remove from oven, transfer to cooling rack and eat when cool. Makes 30 biscuits.

KIRSTY WADE
Winner of 3 Commonwealth Gold Medals

Easy-Peasy Slices

Ingredients

4oz self-raising flour
4oz caster sugar
2 eggs
2oz flaked almonds
Grated lemon rind
A little cinnamon

Method

Mix and cream the flour, sugar and eggs with grated lemon rind. Grease 2 Swiss roll tins. Spread mixture into tins, scatter almonds all over, then sprinkle on some caster sugar and cinnamon. Pop into heated oven at 190°C/375°F (gas mark 5) for 10 or so minutes. Slice into fingers.

MAVIS NICHOLSON

Brack Bread

Ingredients

1 cupful tea
1lb mixed dried fruit
1 cupful brown sugar
2 cupfuls self-raising flour
1 egg, well beaten

Method

Soak the dried fruit and brown sugar overnight in the tea. Next day, add the flour and egg to the soaked mixture. Mix well. Place in a well greased small loaf tin (approx 9″ × 5″ × 3″ deep). Bake for 2 hours on middle shelf at 160°C/300°F (gas mark 2). Take out and leave for 24 hours. To serve slice thinly and spread with butter.

Comments

This is a recipe much used in our family when our children were younger. It is so simple to make even children could make it and ours frequently did so. It is a teabread that keeps quite well and is delicious spread with butter and topped with sliced cheese or conserve – or if you hail from the North both!

THE BARONESS BLATCH, CBE
The House of Lords

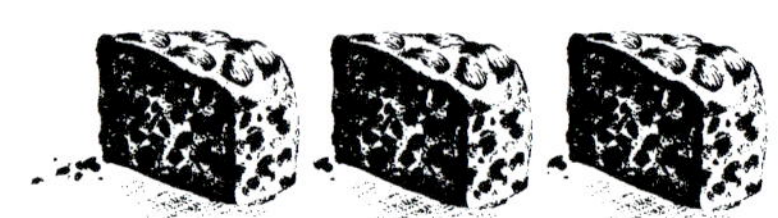

Sweeties

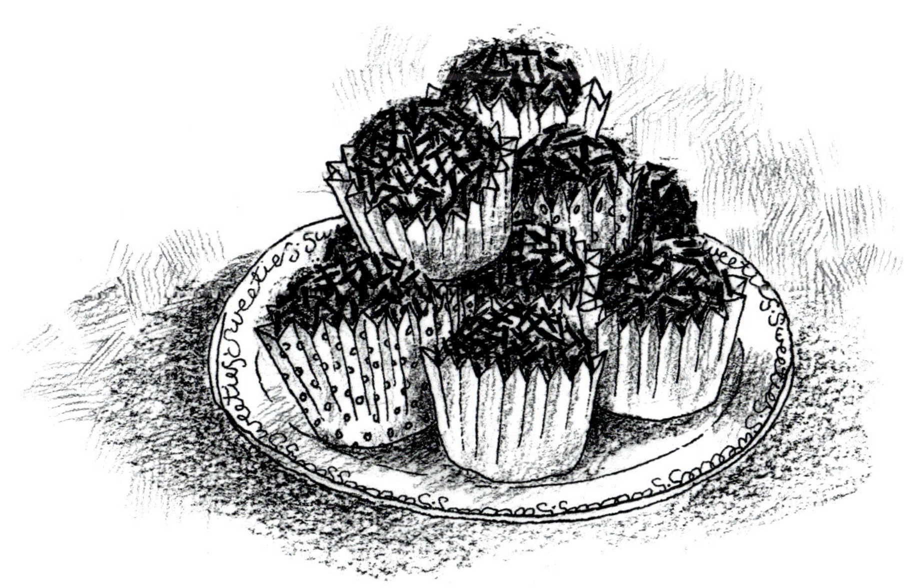

Easy 'No Cook' Truffles

Ingredients

3½oz margarine
2oz oats
3½oz caster sugar
Vanilla essence
1 tablespoon cold strong coffee
2 tablespoons cocoa
Chocolate strands – for coating

Method

Cream margarine and sugar. Add rest of ingredients. Mix well. Roll into balls (about 1 dessertspoon) each and coat with chocolate strands. Place in individual petit four cases.

MRS ROY CASTLE

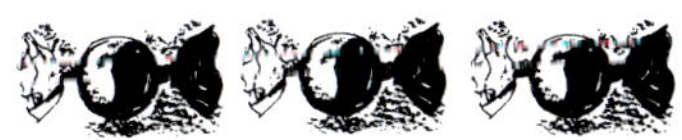

Pseudo Phudge

Ingredients

4oz caster sugar
4oz butter
2oz broken plain chocolate
1 egg
8oz shortcake biscuits, crushed

Method

Melt caster sugar and butter in pan. Add chocolate – or what you like: vanilla essence, 2 tablespoons coffee and/or (my favourite) chopped marshmallows. Beat egg and add. Allow mixture to thicken over low heat. Add biscuit crumbs to mixture and stir well. Pack into greased tin and leave for at least 24 hours before turning out.

Comments

The recipe for this stuff was found when I was going through a mass of cookery books and papers in search of exotic things to please a very dear wife while that was still possible. I had to learn to cook from scratch, of course, and was unable to call on her expertise.

PHIL DAY
Norwich

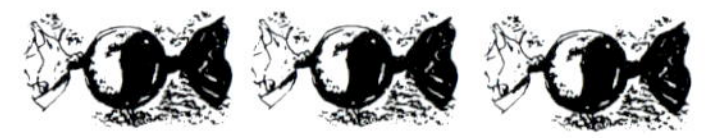

Rum Truffles

Ingredients

2oz melted butter
2oz icing sugar
Dessert spoon cocoa
6oz cake crumbs
Few chopped nuts and cherries
Drop of rum to taste

Method

Blend all ingredients together. Take amounts about the size of ping pong balls and roll in vermicelli. Decorate if desired with piece of cherry or nut, and put into small baking cases.

Comments

Chief Fire Officer Elton's favourite recipe as supplied by his wife.

T. F. ELTON
Tyne & Wear Fire Brigade

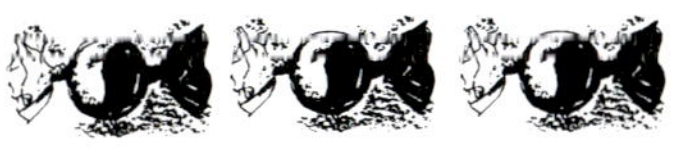

Home-Made Mints

Ingredients

2 cups granulated sugar
½ teaspoon peppermint essence
$^{2}/_{3}$ cup water
Pinch of cream of tartar

Method

Place sugar and water in a saucepan and when it comes to the boil add cream of tartar. Boil without stirring till mixture forms a soft ball. Remove from heat. Place saucepan in cold water then add peppermint and stir in until thick. When cool enough to handle, knead with hands and cut into small rounds. Store in a tin.

DOREEN HALL

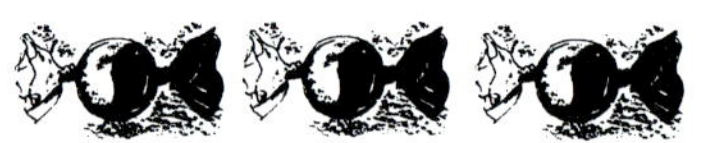

Preserves & Sauces

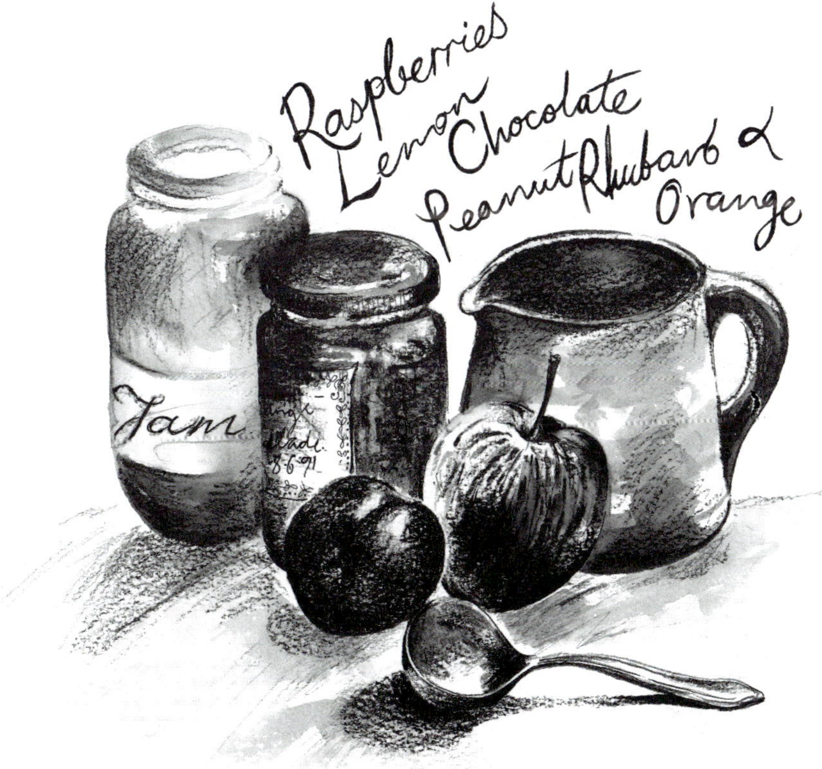

Fresh Lemon Curd

Ingredients

3oz caster sugar
1 large juicy lemon (grated rind and juice)
2 large eggs
2oz unsalted butter

Method

Place grated lemon rind and sugar in bowl. In another bowl whisk lemon juice together with eggs, then pour over the sugar. Add butter cut into little pieces and place the bowl over a pan of barely simmering water. Stir frequently till thickened, about 20 minutes. Cool the curd and use it to sandwich sponges together. Makes enough to sandwich a layer cake. Larger quantities can be made and stored in warmed jam jars. Does not keep for more than about 2-3 weeks.

VI WRIGHT
National Office, Alzheimer's Disease Society, Balham

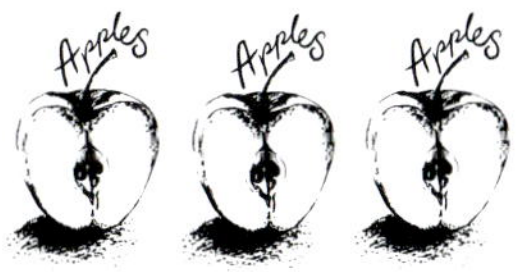

Quince Jelly

Ingredients

4lb quinces
Sugar
6 pints water

Method

Wash quinces well. Cut them up and put into pan with water. Bring to boil and simmer gently for about an hour, or until fruit is clear and tender. Strain through a jelly bag or muslin. To each pint of the juice add 12oz of sugar. Stir well until dissolved then continue to boil the quince jelly rapidly until setting point is reached. Pot and cover.

ROMFORD & BRENTWOOD SUPPORT GROUP

Grape & Almond Mincemeat

Ingredients

1lb muscat grapes
8oz shelled almonds
8oz raisins
4oz sultanas
4oz currants
3 large oranges
6 tablespoons brandy
¼ teaspoon ground cinnamon
All-spice
Whole nutmeg

Method

No fat, no cooking. Skin and seed and chop grapes. Chop the almonds and blend all the ingredients together. Leave to stand for 48 hours. Should fill 4 jars.

PAULINE PENFOLD
Carer

Rhubarb & Orange Chutney

Ingredients

2½lb rhubarb
2 fairly big oranges
3 skinned and chopped onions
1½ pints malt vinegar
2lb demerara sugar
1lb seedless raisins (chopped) or sultanas

Method

Wash and chop rhubarb. Peel and shred oranges after squeezing the juice out. Add juice to the rhubarb. Add the finely shredded orange peel and pulp (pith removed). Add the onions, sugar, raisins (or sultanas) and vinegar. Bring to the boil and simmer for 1½ hours until reduced.

PEGGIE PENROSE
Wokingham Carers' Support Group

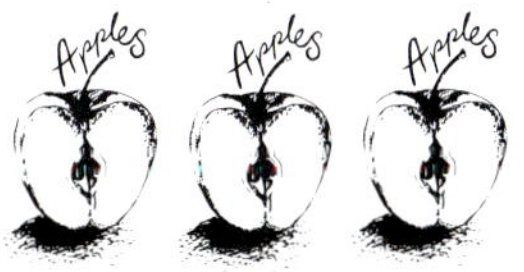

Renee's Raspberry Preserve

Ingredients

4lb raspberries

5lb sugar

Method

Place the fruit in a fire-proof dish in the oven preheated to 'hot' with the sugar in another dish. Leave until both are thoroughly hot (not boiling). Add the sugar to the fruit and beat well until dissolved. Pot up in warmed jars and seal down at once.

Comments

This jam will keep for any length of time, does not need refrigeration and has the flavour of freshly gathered fruit. It is easily made and there is no boiling or simmering, so no weight loss. Loganberries can also be used.

LORNA S. RAYNER
Bideford Branch

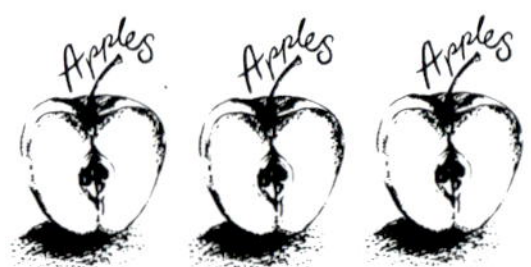

Chunky Orange Marmalade

Ingredients

4lb Seville oranges
2lb sweet oranges
2lb lemons
6 pints water
6lb sugar

Method

Wash fruit thoroughly. Put in a large pan with water and simmer slowly until tender enough to pierce with a fork. This takes approximately one hour. Take off heat and allow to cool.

Remove the fruit, but leave the water in the pan. Cut each piece of fruit into about 8 pieces, then shred each across into thin strips – not too fine or the marmalade will not be chunky.

Discard all the pips. Return the cut up fruit and all the juice, which may have run whilst cutting, to the pan with the water in which the oranges were cooked. Stir in the sugar, bring to the boil, simmer moderately fast, until a little of it will set when tested. Pot whilst hot.

PENELOPE KEITH

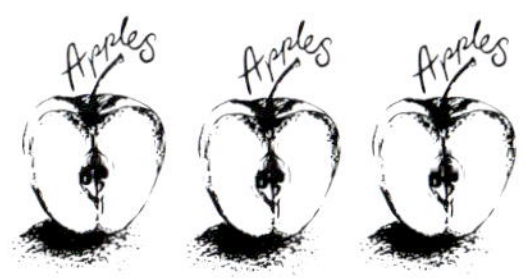

Lemon Sauce

Ingredients

1 large lemon, skin unblemished
2oz butter or margarine
¾ pint (or more) milk
1 heaped tablespoon plain flour

Method

Grate the rind from the lemon, using the small holes of a cheese grater. Retain the rind. Cut the rindlesss lemon in half, and extract the juice on a lemon squeezer. Retain the juice.

Make a white sauce. Make a roux with the melted butter and the flour, and add the milk gradually, stirring constantly.

Add the lemon rind and juice to the sauce. Keep stirring at simmering point. The sauce will thicken very quickly. Add more milk as desired, still stirring.

Comments

This recipe is an invention of my wife Sue. It has proved very popular with many friends, in this country and throughout the world. The sauce goes very well with fish and white meat, or as a dressing for asparagus, new potatoes and similar vegetables.

STEPHEN SMALLEY
Dean of Chester

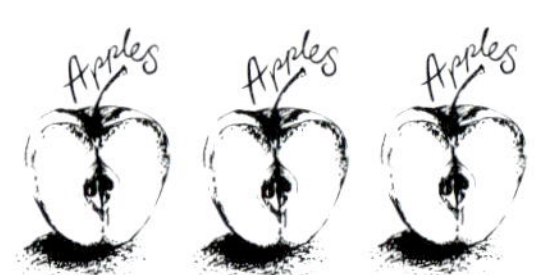

Sauce for Cold Chicken

Ingredients

2 tablespoons clear honey
2 teaspoons curry powder
7 teaspoons mango chutney
½ pint mayonnaise (Hellmans)
¼ pint double cream

Method

Combine all ingredients and coat chicken

SIR MICHAEL SHAW, JP, DL, MP

Cumberland Rum Butter

Ingredients

8oz soft brown sugar
2 tablespoons rum
6oz butter
Grated nutmeg to taste (optional)

Method

Roll brown sugar between two sheets of grease-proof paper to ensure there are no lumps. Put into a bowl with the nutmeg. Melt the butter (do not boil). Pour onto the sugar and nutmeg. Stir well with wooden spoon. Add rum. Stir until well blended and smooth in texture. Pour into a china bowl and allow to set. Serve spread on scones or biscuits. A North Country method traditionally served at Christenings.

PENRITH SUPPORT GROUP

Gado Gado

(INDONESIAN PEANUT SAUCE FOR SALAD)

Ingredients

1 medium-sized onion, minced
2 cloves garlic, minced
5oz peanut butter
2 teaspoons dark soy sauce
1 tablespoon dark brown sugar
2 teaspoons chilli powder
½ teaspoon salt
1 teaspoon instant tamarind (from Chinese grocers)
3 bay leaves
3 tablespoons oil
1 fresh red chilli, finely chopped
¾ cup thick coconut milk (made by dissolving creamed coconut in hot water)

Method

Fry onion, garlic, peanut butter, soy sauce, brown sugar, chilli powder, salt, tamarind and bay leaves in oil for 5 minutes. Add coconut milk and red chilli and simmer till thick and aromatic.

Comments

Serve with a selection or all of the following: bean sprouts, raw carrots, shredded white cabbage, tomatoes, French beans, new potatoes, cucumber and lettuce.

JOHN KEADY

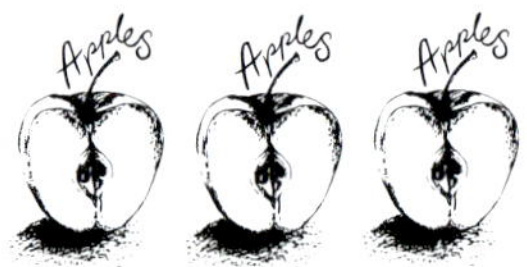

Neapolitan Tomato Sauce

Ingredients

5 cans peeled tomatoes
2-3 cloves garlic, peeled and sliced
1 medium-sized onion, sliced
1 carrot, peeled and sliced
Oil
2-3 sticks celery
Salt and pepper to taste
2 teaspoons brown sugar
2 teaspoons basil leaves, if available

Method

Fry the garlic and chopped onion in 1 tablespoon of oil until soft. Add the tins of tomatoes and then the chopped carrot and cut up celery. Bring to the boil and then simmer for about an hour or until the tomatoes are reduced and quite thick and pulpy. Add salt and pepper and one teaspoon or so of sugar and the basil leaves. Pass the sauce through a sieve or a moulinex machine and it is ready to use.

Comments

This sauce takes a bit of practice but it's worth it!

LYNDA BELLINGHAM

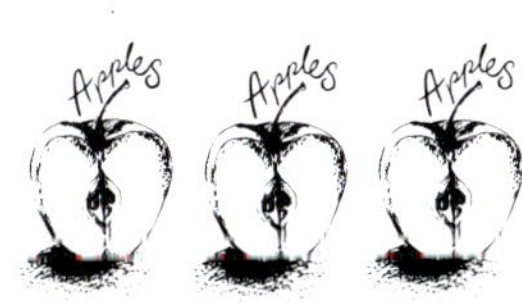

Chocolate Spread – 1

Ingredients

2oz melted plain chocolate, cooled
2oz Stork margarine
1 level tablespoon golden syrup or black treacle

Method

Beat all the ingredients together.

Chocolate Spread – 2

Ingredients

¼ pint milk
1 dessert spoon flour
2 dessertspoons sugar
3 dessertspoons cocoa

Method

Blend flour, cocoa and sugar with a little milk. Pour over rest of milk, When boiling, return to the pan and stir until smooth and thick. Use when cold.

MARY HEDDINGTON
Dartford Branch

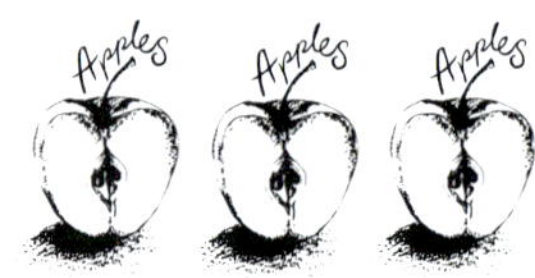

Drinks & Dips

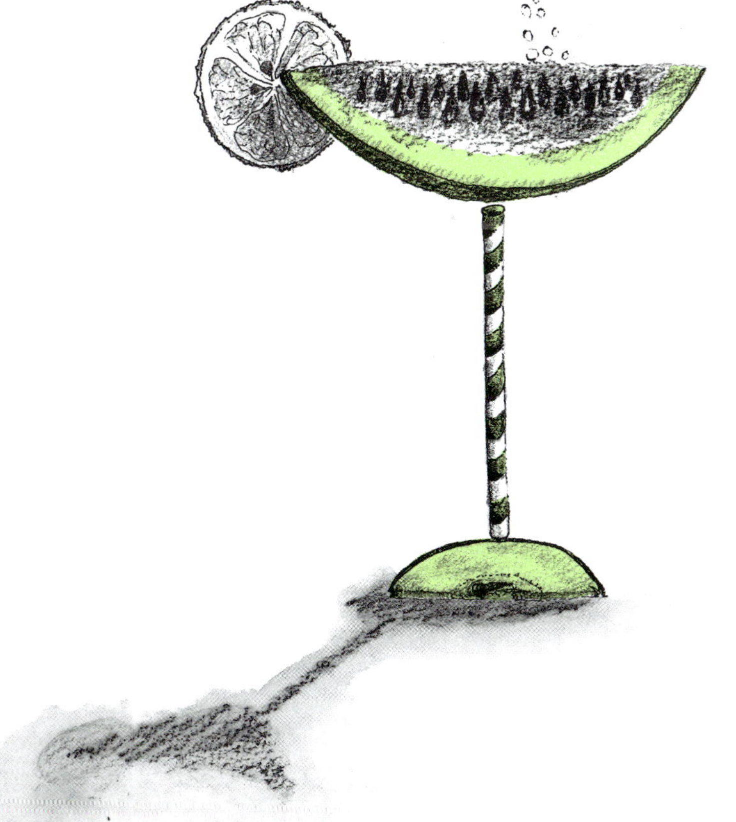

Irish Cream Whisky

Ingredients

14oz tin condensed milk
1 small tin evaporated milk
1 cup hot water
Coffee granules
1 teaspoon gelatine
1 teaspoon vanilla essence
1 cup whisky, rum or brandy

Method

Make a cup of coffee with the granules and hot water. Mix with gelatine in a bowl. Add condensed milk, evaporated milk and vanilla essence. Whisk together well or blend in liquidiser. Add whisky, then whisk again before bottling. Should be ready to drink in twelve hours.

MARY CALLAND
Rhyl & District Branch

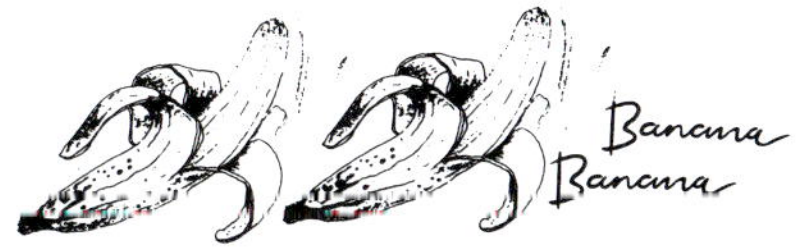

Home-Made Orange/Lemon Squash

Ingredients

4 lemons
4 oranges
4lb granulated sugar
4 pints boiling water
2oz citric acid (from chemist)
1oz tartaric acid (from chemist)
½oz Epsom salts (from chemist)

Method

Wash fruit. Boil water. Put sugar in large basin and pour boiling water over it: stir to dissolve. Add acids and Epsom salts and continue stirring until all dissolved. Cut rind of fruit finely with sharp knife or peeler. Cut fruit in halves and squeeze roughly. Add everything except pith to the syrup.

Leave to soak for 24 hours, stirring occasionally. Sieve and bottle. Keep in fridge and dilute in normal way. This recipe makes enough for about 4½ squash bottles.

H. W. ACWORTH
Oxfordshire Branch

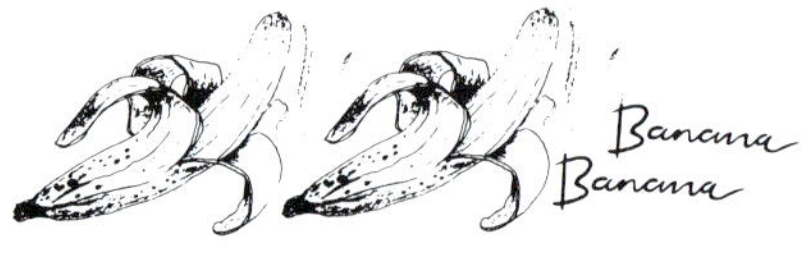

White Wine Punch

Ingredients

1 bottle Sauterne wine
½ pint lemonade
½ lemon
1 tablespoon lime juice cordial
2oz maraschino cherries
Some sprigs of mint

Method

Slice the lemon and cut each slice into quarters. Put in a jug or bowl and pour over the wine. Add the lime juice cordial and mint. Drain the cherries and add them.

Allow to stand. Just before serving, add the lemonade and, if required, some ice.

Comments

This can be tried with other wines and in larger quantities for parties.

A. FRANKLIN

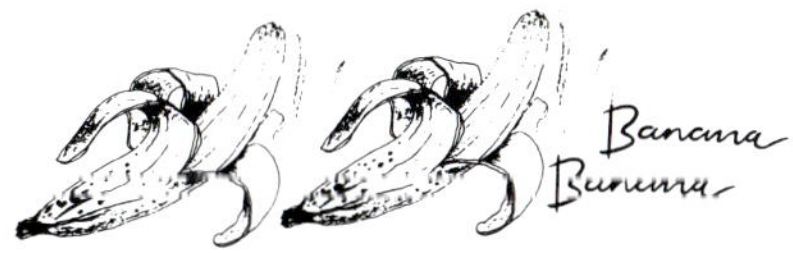

Banana Milk Shake

Ingredients

1 banana
2 scoops ice cream
1 pint milk
1 rounded tablespoon (1oz) sugar

Method

Peel the banana, place in a bowl and mash with a fork. Add sugar and milk and whisk until frothy. Pour into glasses and stir in a scoop of ice cream until almost dissolved.

Serves 2

JOANNE KEARSLEY

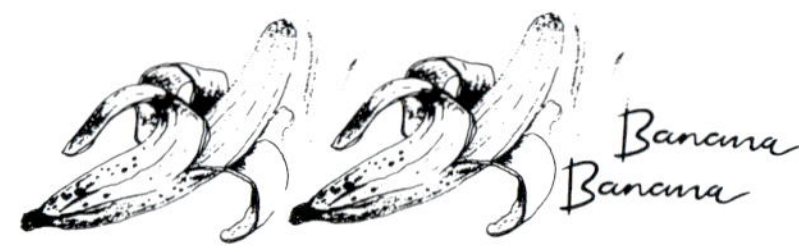

Pink Gin

Ingredients

5-10 drops Angostura bitters (according to taste)
1 part dry gin
2-2½ parts ice cold water

Method

For 1 glass: Put the bitters in a wine glass (not a sherry glass). Swirl the bitters to spread around the sides. Add the gin and water. Swirl until the bitters mix. Drink.

Comments

CHEERS!

KURT LAND
Poole & District Branch

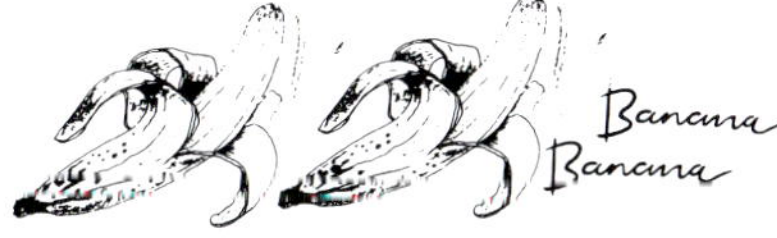

Cheese Dip

Ingredients

4-6oz low fat cream cheese
2 flat tablespoons pumpkin seed
2-3 teaspoons capers
Several shakes of Worcester sauce
Cream to thin

Method

Grind pumpkin seed in 'Magimix' or liquidiser. Add cream cheese, capers and mix. Add cream or top of the milk to obtain the required consistency.

MARTIN MUNCASTER

Stilton Dip

Ingredients

8oz Stilton cheese
4oz cream cheese
4 tablespoons milk
4 pickled onions, finely chopped

Method

Cream cheeses until well blended. Beat in milk. Stir chopped pickled onions into cheese mixture. Season with salt and pepper and serve with a tasty brown bread.

CHRISTINE WHILD
Oxfordshire

Index

Index

Index

Index

Index

VEGETARIAN AND VEGETABLE DISHES